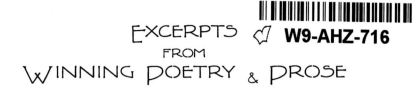

EXCERPTS
FROM
WINNING POETRY & PROSE

SHE PARES THE APPLES WITH BLUE FIRE IN HER BLADE,
SWIPES THE PEELS INTO THE BAG BEFORE THE PILE BUILDS,
PLUNGES THE KNIFE INTO WHITE FLESH, PEELS AND PEELS.

SHE DID THE DOUGH YESTERDAY, POUNDED IT INTO THE
REQUISITE BALL, SLAMMING IT ON THE COUNTER, EACH
THWACK A DRUM ROLL AND TRUMPET CALL. IT DOESN'T

MATTER HOW SWEET THE CINNAMON, HOW THE DARK BROWN
SUGAR SOFTENS HER SHAKING HANDS AND SHE WATCHES IT
FALL BETWEEN THE APPLE PIECES FINDING RESTING PLACES

IN THE SHADOWS WAITING FOR HEAT AND BUTTER TO START
RAISING A SCENT SHE CAN LIVE WITH, 14 YEARS OF SOAP PADS
AND SCOURING POWDER HAVING TURNED HER TO STONE.

FROM JUST DESSERTS
BY MICHELE F. COOPER

THE WAITRESS RETURNED TO FILL MY CUP THREE-QUARTERS FULL WITH THE LAST BIT
OF COFFEE FROM A GLASS POT. I RAISED THE CUP TO MY LIPS AND BLEW ON IT FOR
A FEW SECONDS BEFORE TAKING A SIP. IT WAS STRONG AND VERY COLD. I WAVED THE
WAITRESS BACK OVER.

"WHAT'CHA NEED, DARLIN'?"

"MY COFFEE IS COLD," I TOLD HER.

SHE GLANCED DOWN AT MY CUP. "WELL, YOU'RE JUST GOING TO HAVE TO DRINK
IT A LITTLE FASTER NOW, AREN'T YOU?" SHE GRABBED A STEAMING POT FROM THE
HOT PLATE BEHIND HER AND FILLED THE REMAINING QUARTER-CUP. "THERE YOU GO,
NICE AND WARM." SHE THEN FILLED THE CUP OF THE GENTLEMAN SITTING NEXT TO ME.
"YOUR PLATE'LL BE RIGHT UP, WALTER."

"EXCUSE ME," I SAID, GAINING HER ATTENTION AGAIN. "YOU THINK I COULD GET
ANOTHER CUP OF COFFEE?"

"TO GO?" SHE SAID.

I RAISED MY CUP. "ANOTHER CUP. A HOT CUP?"

"WHY, YOU HAVEN'T EVEN DRANK THAT ONE YET." SHE CHUCKLED AND MOVED
ON DOWN THE COUNTER OFFERING MORE HOT REFILLS.

FROM SUNNY SIDE UP
BY KEVIN WATSON

OTHER BOOKS BY WHITNEY SCOTT

A KISS IS STILL A KISS
ALTERNATIVES – ROADS LESS TRAVELLED
DANCING TO THE END OF THE SHINING BAR
EARTH BENEATH, SKY BEYOND
FEATHERS, FINS & FUR – ANIMAL STORIES
FREEDOM'S JUST ANOTHER WORD
LISTEN TO THE MOON
PRAIRIE HEARTS – WOMEN VIEW THE MIDWEST
WORDS AGAINST THE SHIFTING SEASONS

TAKE TWO –
THEY'RE SMALL

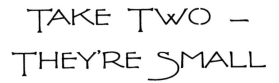

EDITED & DESIGNED
BY
WHITNEY SCOTT

OUTRIDER PRESS, INC.

CRETE, ILLINOIS

TAKE TWO - THEY'RE SMALL IS PUBLISHED BY OUTRIDER
PRESS IN AFFILIATION WITH THE TALLGRASS WRITERS GUILD.

CHOCOLATE BAR BY MAUREEN CONNOLLY ORIGINALLY APPEARED IN
HAMMERS NUMBER 8, 1994

THE DIET BY CJ LAITY ORIGINALLY APPEARED IN BEST OF TOMORROW, 1992

'FOOD THAT RIDES OFF INTO THE SUNSET" BY LYNN VEACH SADLER
WON ROBERT RUARK FOUNDATION'S 1996 POETRY COMPETITION AND '98
HONORABLE MENTION AWARDS, THE LONE WOLF REVIEW, 1998.

A SHORTER VERSION OF ROSEMARY SERLUCA'S "PASS THE PASTA..." WAS
ORIGINALLY PUBLISHED IN THE CHRISTIAN SCIENCE MONITOR, 12/98

"EGGPLANT" BY LISA SORNBERGER WAS ORIGINALLY PUBLISHED IN NEW
VIRGINIA REVIEW.

"THE UNBEARABLE WEIGHT OF EMPTY" BY BEVERLY SWEET, R.N.
ORIGINALLY APPEARED IN MEDHUNTERS WINTER 2001

MEMORIES FROM THE HEARTH BY DIANALEE VELIE ORIGINALLY APPEARED
IN GRANDMOTHER'S TABLE

THE QUEEN BEE BY TAMMY WILSON ORIGINALLY APPEARED IN
BRANCHES 2000

BOOK DESIGN & PRODUCTION
BY
WHITNEY SCOTT

TRADEMARKS AND BRAND NAMES
HAVE BEEN PRINTED IN INITIAL
CAPITAL LETTERS

ONCE AGAIN
FOR
DR. MARIA ISABELLA BROWN

TABLE OF CONTENTS

2ND PLACE PROSE

HON. MENTION PROSE

3RD PLACE POETRY

1ST PLACE POETRY

INTRODUCTION

 at. Live. It's so basic. Without food, we die. Food sustains life. Yet food, as well as the provider of energy necessary to maintain life, is also a potent transmitter – of love, of ethnic culture and identity, and of memories. Perhaps most of all, memories.

We may bake a loved one's favorite chocolate cake to better say "I love you." Many believe such symbols are far more meaningful than words, and for that matter, many see in chocolate more power than they ascribe to most things, including words.

We take pride in a table spread with our own ethnic specialities made from scratch (of course!) with authentic ingredients bought, perhaps, from a tiny deli in "the old neighborhood." And if no one serving us in that deli speaks English, so much the better, for the resulting dishes sing more passionately of their history and heritage – and of our own. Heritage helps form our identity, helps us know who we are, and where we fit – whether in a national multicultural society, a neighborhood, or a family.

From food comes our earliest memories of the most elemental nourishment, from infants' milk to children's discoveries of solid sustenance. Memory, like heritage, affirms our sense of self, and recollections of the foods that helped shape us physically, emotionally, and spiritually continue to nourish and nurture us throughout life.

Naturally, we are driven to write about this multi-faceted life force that goes straight to the heart of our being – of who we are, where we're from, and where we want to be. Just as naturally, we want to share the passion, sweetness, sorrow, and joy found in the food that is before us now, and found in our memories of food from times past – the stuff that so many dreams are made of.

WHITNEY SCOTT
APRIL, 2002

MRS. SHEELEY'S COLE SLAW

BY TIMOTHY AMSDEN

Not creamy but tart and sweet and clear,
a simple bright salad that holds cabbage
and onion and summer memories crisp
in touches of celery and mustard.

I never knew Mrs. Sheeley. She
cared for Lucia and Linda's children
decades ago, a white-haired aproned
unflappable care giver and slaw master.

With her perfect recipe she is famous.
Unlike the bold renown of a poet,
Mrs. Sheeley's fame is grains so small
they sift through cracks and
lodge in lives, recipe cards riffling
into recipe boxes like slow snow.

MRS. SHEELEY'S COLE SLAW

1 MEDIUM HEAD CABBAGE
1 LARGE ONION
3/4 CUP SUGAR

DRESSING:
3/4 CUP SALAD OIL
1 CUP WHITE VINEGAR
1 TEASPOON EACH CELERY SEED, DRY MUSTARD, SUGAR
1 AND 1/2 TEASPOONS SALT

SHRED CABBAGE, CHOP ONION, LAYER CABBAGE, ONION, SUGAR IN BOWL. COMBINE ALL DRESSING INGREDIENTS EXCEPT OIL AND BRING TO BOIL. ADD OIL AND BRING TO BOIL. POUR HOT DRESSING OVER SLAW AND REFRIGERATE. DRAIN OFF MOST OF THE EXCESS DRESSING AS YOU TRANSFER SLAW TO SERVING BOWL.

BALM

BY TIMOTHY AMSDEN

Every night I place a glass of water beside my bed.
At midnight I wake, grope and swallow
balm to a mouth gaped pasty with sleep.

What trust is this, to blindly ingest water long sat in an open glass
in a dark room with desert insects who also perhaps seek wet;
who may find their end in my glass of water,
in the damp and deadly trap beside my bed?

Some night perhaps my blind gulp will include
a weakly stroking beetle,
ridged carapace just right to bind
itself to my sticky throat
and be expelled by a rough cough
which startles us all
awake.

Or some fat, soft-bodied thing
will slip down with the water,
a dead gob of insect,
waking us with my
after-the-fact
frisson.

A less trusting man would cover his glass and avoid
these night adventures, but then perhaps
water-lusting insects
would seek other oases and find
the mouth,
slack jawed with sleep,
moist and redolent with dinner gases,
a red meat cave of delights,
easy pickings for the bug
with a commitment
to do a little
digging.

TO EAT FROSTING OFF THE BEATER *

BY ELLEN WADE BEALS

Be bowlside when the icing is ready.

Hold the beater like a lollipop.

Start with first silver arc.

Use tongue to lick sweetness from the exterior.

When frosting from first arc is gone,
twirl beater to next one.

Continue until all frosting is licked
from outside of all arcs.

Use a similar procedure
on interior sides.

To reach the inside top,
that flat disc where the arcs meet,
try to poke your tongue
in between.

You will not get it all.

Rinse.
Repeat with other beater.

NOTE: THESE DIRECTIONS MAY ALSO APPLY TO MASHED POTATOES.
*GENERAL ELECTRIC PORTABLE MIXER MODELS 22 & M24

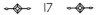

TILLING AND DRILLING

BY DONNA L. BLACK

heat gives me heartburn. Always has. I ate a lot of it when wheat was the new hot diet thing. Wheat bread, crackers, pasta – anything with wheat in it. Had me some hefty heartburn until I finally figured it out. That's why I can't believe I'm standin' in this wheat field checkin' out the wheat to see if it's ready for harvest.

Sam says, "Soon...I think. Maybe."

He grew up on this farm. Ran away, sort of, when he went away to college. Swore he'd never come back. Went into video camera work after graduation and loved it.

One night, the food expert he was filming for the TV news spot that night – choked to death in the restaurant. Closed the restaurant right down for a couple of weeks, we heard later. Best tape Sam ever made, too.

Now, talk about coincidence: that same night Sam's folks called and begged him to come home. Seems his brother got caught robbing the local liquor store. The folks would need Sam to help with the farm until Jason got out of jail. They were in their forties when he and Jason were born, and couldn't manage the place on their own anymore. Sam sent back money all the time, but didn't go home, except to visit now and again.

Sam woke me pounding on my door. It was after midnight, for Pete's sake. When I let him in he grabbed my hand, half dragged me to the couch, sat me down, fell on his knees and with desperation in his voice said, "Elly, I love you! Marry me now...please." Said he wasn't goin' back to that farm by himself and he sure as hell wasn't gonna leave me here by myself.

I was the copy girl at the station and not bad lookin', if I do say so myself. My red hair was a little carroty for my taste, but Sam liked it. All my parts were well stacked and in excellent workin' order, but I seemed to be havin' trouble with my hearing.

I gotta admit, he threw me for a minute. I just stared at him. I gazed at his gorgeous, curly brown hair (the kind you can't keep your fingers out of) and wondered why men always have longer, fuller eyelashes than women do. "What farm?" I managed to croak.

Before he could answer, I realized what he had just said...asked...wanted...ME, he wanted ME! My response was not totally dignified as I whooped with joy, "Yes! Yes! I love you! I love you! Yes! I'll marry you! Yes!" I dropped down next to him. "What farm?"

We got hitched by a justice of the peace and left for Kansas. New York to Kansas...made me nervous. Sam said it was like doin' the rainbow thing backwards, instead of going over it...we were going under it. That, of course, reassured me no end.

We hadn't told his parents about me. Sam said we'd surprise them. The closer we got, the less sure I was, though. I mean what with Jason in jail and all, maybe they'd had enough surprises lately. So we called them from Indiana and said we were married. They were sure nice about it, but I could tell they were nervous about me and I can't say I blamed them. I was nervous about them too, and the farm, and Sam going home when I knew he didn't want to.

He had just started getting recognition for his work in New York. But Sam said he felt obligated to go back because he'd left and stuck Jason with the farm, and maybe that's why his kid brother got in trouble in the first place. I thought that was nuts, but didn't say so. The weather turned extra nasty as we got near the place. We pulled into the farmyard just as the heavens opened and torrents of water came rushing down. The wind was screaming, thunder and lightning were shaking the ground like crazy, and by the time we got to the porch, we were drenched.

The house was open, but there no one was home. Then we heard the roaring – like a train. Sam didn't say a word, just grabbed my hand and dashed out the back door. I had seen his face so I didn't ask why we were going outside. I raced with him and we scrambled into their storm shelter. Sam had one hell of a time gettin' that door down, but it finally closed.

After awhile, it got quiet. We opened the door and peeked out. The rain was falling gently now and the wind had died down. The tornado was gone, and the house looked fine. The barn, too. Then Sam saw the silo was gone.

Later the cops came. Turns out Sam's folks must have got caught outside in the storm and run into the silo. Cops said they found the silo with his parents still in it about two miles down on the next farm. It was standin' up straight and all, and looked like it belonged there, but his folks were both gone; shuffled off their mortal coil; joined their ancestors; you know...deceased. His mom was still hangin' on to an umbrella and his dad was still holdin' her hand. *Not* an auspicious beginning to our homecoming.

Funny thing was, the tornado never did touch the wheat field. It came down and took the silo and the tractor. At least we figure it took the tractor 'cause it was gone.

The wheat was beat down some, but mostly was undisturbed. We never did find that tractor.

◇ ◇ ◇

After the funeral, we drove down to see Jason. He asked us to keep the farm goin' for him. Said he really liked farming and wanted to get back to it when he got out. He'd just got in with a bad crowd. "You know, kid stuff," he said. Sam reminded him he'd be 30 when he got out in two years; it wasn't kid stuff, for God's sake.

Sam said we'd think about it.

By the time we got back to the farm he said we'd try it for one growin' season, if I agreed. If it didn't work we'd "cut and run" back to New York; if it did work, we'd stick it out and wait for Jason. I said it sounded like a damn fine idea to me. It didn't really, but I knew this was something Sam needed to do, so I said it was a damn fine idea.

Wow! The things you don't know. You don't know you don't know them until you need to know them and you find out you don't know them after all. We spent most of our time learning about wheat. The "tilling" (preparation of land for planting) and the "drilling" (what the farmers call the actual planting) had been done. The farmer next door (the one who inherited the silo and who, by the way, had the patience of a saint) said the crop would be ready to harvest in late June or early July probably, depending on the weather. So we started readin' and talkin' to Jason and some guy from the Farm Bureau.

It was March, and we needed to know how and when and what by June. It was a nightmare of not knowing. Back when Sam had left for college they'd grown corn and had cows. Then Jason had talked his folks into planting wheat and getting rid of the cows. I personally was thrilled the cows were gone.

Wheat can get sick. Who knew? It gets Leaf Rust, Smut, Streak Mosaic, Barley Yellow Dwarf, and if that's not enough, it gets eaten by Greenbugs, Russian Wheat Aphids, Hessian Flies, Cutworms, etc. It's drowned by too much rain, choked by weeds, smashed by hail and strong winds, and keels over or refuses to grow if it doesn't get enough water or nutrients.

Jason talked his folks into planting wheat; so tell me: what was he thinking?

We found out that our wheat was seed wheat for farmers to plant, or "drill." The wheat has to be harvested after the plant has died and the grain is hard and dry, but before the plants fall over or the grains start fallin' out of their heads. Egad!

Speaking of heads, mine is over full and Sam says his brain is twirlin' like a Tasmanian Devil. Oh! One more thing; after you harvest with the Combine (the farmer next door came over and reacquainted Sam with the machine) you have to send the wheat to the seed cleaner at an Elevator before you can load it into the bins.

Oh, man! Whatever was Jason thinking?

Believe it or not, by mid-June we finally got a handle on all this, thanks to our next door neighbor, Jason, and the Farm Bureau. So that's how I'm standin' in this field and thinking, *Yep! This is gonna work.*

Never think you have it all together. Fate always steps in — laughin' the whole way.

◇ ◇ ◇

I can't sleep. Sam is snorin' away next to me, so I get up and go out onto the back porch. It's a nice, warm night with a gorgeous breeze. I figure it's after midnight, and sit on the porch swing to commune with the stars for awhile.

I look up at the heavens when lights out over the wheat field catch my eye. I see two balls of white light dancin' over the wheat. Within an instant they become motionless. There is no sound.

From somewhere, I get a shot of either bravery or stupidity and I leap off the porch and begin to run toward the lights. As I get closer, I feel cracklin' in the air, like just before lightning strikes close by. I hear a whooshing sound and I'm close enough to see the sudden movement in the wheat as if a great wind has swooped down.

I freeze as this jet of hot air sweeps across me and the two balls of light disappear; then silence again.

Man! I gotta say I'm freaked. I dash back to the house and tear upstairs and wake Sam – who tells me I'm dreamin' or crazy and grumbles, "Go back to bed."

I get back in bed, but I know what I saw.

◊ ◊ ◊

I must have dozed off 'cause the next thing I heard was the alarm. Sam was already shavin' and I ran and looked out the bedroom window. You could see the wheat field from our bedroom and in the center of the field the wheat looked flattened or maybe gone.

"Sam, darling!" I cooed at him, "Come look at this and then tell me I was dreamin' or crazy."

"Shit!" he bellowed when he saw and grabbed his shirt and ran down the stairs. I watched him dash out the back door.

I threw on my clothes and followed him to the barn. When I got to there, he was on the roof. "It looks like some kind of design," he shouted. "Call and get somebody out here. I want to know what the hell is goin' on."

Fate! That's what was goin' on. Seems we had a Crop Circle. I thought Crop Circles only happened in England. Who would have thought the middle of Kansas? Can you believe it? Sam and me never heard anything more exciting in our lives. Even Jason was impressed when we called him. "Can we make any money?" he wanted to know.

Sam told him to "zip it"; but I noticed, as he watched the farm turning into a circus, he'd get this look on his face. "Hmmm," he said thoughtfully more than once.

Sam got me talking to one of the experts who showed up. The man told me our Crop Circle was in a geometric design. The wheat stalks were bent, but not broken. The top layer bent clockwise and the layer under it was counterclockwise. Said they would show us the pictures the helicopter was taking so we could see what the whole thing looked like. Cool.

He also said the wheat seeds would probably have a better nutrient value within the design. Seems that holds true for the wheat in all the designs they had investigated so far. Better wheat – that sounded cool, too.

I walked with him into the design and immediately felt dizzy. He said to stand still for a moment and it would pass. He was right, and after a minute or two I felt amazingly great. He told me most people were affected in some way when they entered the designs.

He said science was still arguin' theories of how the circles formed. Some say microwave radiation, but the fact is no one really knows for sure.

I learned from him that when the winter snow came it would probably melt fastest over the design, even after new tilling and drilling had taken place. He had heard of one farm where geese had been seen splitting their formation rather than fly over the design area. He said the circles had been found in sand, blueberries, even trees, and the formation that bothered him the most was the one that shows the universe without the Earth.

He also told me that almost everyone involved with the Crop Circles feels someone is tryin' to tell us something. "Who?" I said. "Why can't they just tell us?"

"Those two questions," he said, "are the same ones everyone is asking."

Sam and Jason had to decide – did we harvest or did we promote our Crop Circle? Jason said advertise and charge admission. Sam said harvest the grain in the circle when it was time and see if it was a better quality. We wound up doing both.

Sam also made a documentary. We sold it – big time.

So – we made lots of money from that Crop Circle – no heartburn there!

◇ ◇ ◇

Sam and I are here in New York now that Jason's out and back on the farm. I'm happy to be back at the station. Sam decided to go freelance. He can get a shot nobody else even thinks of, much less sees. He is too, too terrific and I adore him.

I kept some of the grain in a tiny bottle that I wear around my neck when life gets bumpy. It makes me feel better. Sam says it's all in my head, but I don't think he really believes that. After all, he kept some, too.

Jason says every season the wheat in the Crop Circle area comes up better and more nutritious than the rest. He's married to a great wife and they have two cool kids – they all love the farm. Sam and I wouldn't trade our time there for anything. The Crop Circle thing was huge, stupendous, but when all is said and done – we're city folks.

BIRDS – NOT OF A FEATHER

BY MARGARET B. BLACKMAN

t's the classic photo ad: the product at eye level thrust at the viewer by two attractive young women. "You want this," their cheesecake smiles tease. Their offering is a cardboard box containing a tofu turkey, or Tofurkey – to be more commodity-precise. One of the alluring hucksters is my vegan daughter; the other, a vegetarian friend she has brought home from college to join us for Thanksgiving. I, out of necessity, not allure, purchased the Tofurkey for them. The Thanksgiving meal for the rest of us, a 23-pound, freshly killed *Meleagris gallopavo* was roasting in the oven as I snapped their photo.

A few months before Thanksgiving, just as I had grown comfortable with her dedicated vegetarianism, my daughter confessed that she'd gone vegan on me. She was no longer eating eggs or any dairy products. Two years ago her high school foray into vegetarianism had created its own crisis when her hands turned blue after track practice and she felt faint. Her pediatrician prescribed blood tests and a visit to a pediatric cardiologist to rule out heart problems. Her heart was fine, her blood not so fine, so we were directed to a nutritionist who planned healthy meatless meals and prescribed supplements of Vitamin B-12 and iron. I bought the California Culinary Academy's *Vegetarian Cooking* and the acclaimed *Italian Vegetarian Cookbook*. If my daughter and, occasionally, I must eat vegetarian, we would do it in style. And we did, two or three times a week, taking turns cooking vegetarian meals like Garbanzo Ragout and *Shiitake* Potpie. I didn't mind eating less meat and happily continued even after she left home for college.

Vegetarianism, as a healthful alternative to a meat-heavy diet, dates to 18th century Europe. It arrived in America in the early 19th century intertwined with health reform, morality and religion. The prominent New England Alcott family proselytized the virtues of a vegetable diet, and many famous 20th century vegetarians followed, among them Albert Einstein, Dr. Benjamin Spock, and all four of the Beatles. Nonetheless, as an anthropologist, I know that in the course of human history there has been no culture that is totally vegetarian. Certainly not where I work as a cultural anthropologist and where my daughter spent six summers of her childhood. The Nunamiut Eskimo of northern interior Alaska have never known a vegetarian in their culture. Food to them is "meat." And "meat" is caribou. If you don't have caribou seven days a week, or the occasional mountain sheep, then you eat some of the white man's store-bought meat – chicken, beef, or pork.

We know now that the 19th century vegetarians were right. A vegetarian diet, with careful attention to protein consumption, is healthy. In today's agribusiness world, many argue vegetarianism's virtues: no worry about ingesting antibiotics administered to prevent disease in animals raised in close quarters, no saturated fat like that which marbles the flesh of feedlot stock fattened for slaughter. No high cholesterol, either. No guilt over eating something less than humanely raised. And no more eating from the top of the food chain, but satisfaction in consuming less ecologically costly protein.

Last year at Thanksgiving, my daughter's vegetarianism hardly was noticed. She skipped the turkey and gravy, but relished the stuffing, the whipped potatoes and butter, and the egg-based dinner rolls from the recipe I inherited from my maternal grandmother. This year, in addition to those rolls, I made French bread pure enough for the most fastidious vegan, and I kept the freshly grated parmesan cheese and the anchovy and egg-laced Caesar dressing separate from the romaine lettuce salad. Before mashing the potatoes with half-and-half and butter, I put some aside so that my daughter could whip hers with soy milk and a "trans fat-free" butter substitute. I made a separate batch of stuffing for the two vegetable eaters as well, omitting the Italian sausage, and moistening the herbed bread cubes with vegetable broth. I respectfully baked this alternative stuffing at farthest remove from the turkey with which it was forced to share the oven.

The Tofurkey, spirited off to bake at a neighbor's, came with its own stuffing, a gluey gray-brown mix, unquestionably inferior in taste and texture to either of my stuffings – and Tofurkey "gravy," a thick, dirt-brown concoction in a sealed plastic container. The Thanksgiving vegan meal was filling and contained, in name anyway, all the items that belong to the traditional Thanksgiving feast. But it was clear to me that these veggie munchers and we turkey gobblers were not sharing the same Thanksgiving dinner. And that, to me, was hugely significant and not a little sad.

A roasting turkey creates its own domestic aura. Aromas of crispy fat and cooking meat, filtered through sage-garlic-sausage stuffing, stir the appetite as they tug at memory. Thanksgivings past tumbled through my mind as I chopped vegetables and rolled dough at the kitchen island. Memories came too of winter feasts on a remote island in northern British Columbia where I did my first fieldwork as an anthropologist. The native Haida people there are inveterate feast givers, and turkey, introduced by 19th century English missionaries, is the standard feast food. Before a feast, a dozen or more turkeys are cooked in ovens belonging to members of the host's extended family. Slabs of hot turkey are served up on fine bone china along with stuffing, mashed potatoes, mashed turnips, gravy and cole slaw. The china plates form neat, tight rows on linen-covered feast tables. Days later, whole turkey carcasses, on their way to becoming turkey soup, poke above the rims of stainless steel pots. Steam rises from the simmering pots and condenses on kitchen windows. My Thanksgiving turkey would meet a similar fate, cooked from a recipe given me by my adopted Haida grandmother.

My guests arrived in late afternoon, bearing their own Thanksgiving offerings: A mother's cranberry sauce made with fresh cranberries, apples, oranges and sugar. An okra, spinach, and cheese dish from his island home contributed by my Caribbean boyfriend. Stuffed acorn squashes garnished with freshly grated Parmesan cheese. There was an apartheid about this last dish; two cheeseless, vegan-safe squash rested on a separate baking sheet. We uncorked the wine and gathered in the kitchen, warmed by the roasting turkey that I wrested from the oven every 20 minutes to turn and baste.

The Tofurkey is a recent food product made possible by an ancient method of processing soybeans that originated in the Chou dynasty (1122-246 BC) in China. The fermented bean curd, or tofu, resembles in shape and color a large turkey breast. The unattached "drumsticks" are made from tempeh, another soy product that has a more meat-like texture than the smooth tofu. Unconvincingly patted into flat drumstick shapes, the tempeh could be mistaken for anemic hamburger. The manufacturers had thought of everything. A "slice" of "leftover" Tofurkey, sealed in plastic, was included for the morrow's luncheon sandwich, and most incredulously, a pair of "wishsticks" were similarly preserved in plastic. I surely paid for these extras, because like other vegan products, the Tofurkey is pricey, costing more than the same-sized real thing.

The irony of this nutritious vegetable product is that it is made to look like the very thing its consumers are avoiding – meat. Why should a meatless, vegetable product aimed at vegetarians resemble meat? Can they even morally eat this ersatz animal? That was not a consideration for our Thanksgiving vegetarians. Perhaps, in this case, the animal resemblance is because the turkey is simply so symbolic, because it is such an American icon and a metaphor for this ever-so-American national holiday. I suspect also that the Tofurkey's resemblance to the real thing is an attempt to appease the true meat eaters at the Thanksgiving table, to reassure them that the vegetarians are joining them in spirit if not actually eating flesh.

Thanksgiving has always been my favorite holiday. No gifts to fret over and wrap. Just good food, good company, and good conversation. It's the one day when you are expected to linger in the kitchen and linger at the table. The one day when second helpings and full tummies are de rigueur. "Take, eat, these are my grandmother's rolls, and this, the moistest turkey this side of heaven. The very best turkey I've made in my 30 years of cooking Thanksgiving turkeys." No, thank you, the guests nodded when offered some of the Tofurkey. I refused it too. I hate tofu, and I resent this manufactured avian imposter with no history on this holiday when everyone in America sits down to eat turkey. It has no taste either, as I later discovered.

But veganism is not about taste. You don't become a vegan because you like the cuisine. (I wouldn't even deign to call it "cuisine.") You become a vegan because you think it's a healthier way to live, or because you believe in animal rights, or because you think agribusiness, especially livestock-raising, is raping the land and ruining the environment. You may think all those things even if you don't act politically on them, other than by what you don't eat. Veganism is time-consuming and it spawns its own obsessions – reading labels to look for hidden animal products, perfecting the ability to detect meat-based products in any dish that you're served, scouting out all the restaurants that accommodate vegan diners, learning arcane details about food processing in order to avoid contact with any animal product of any kind. But maybe, as a friend suggested, the bottom line is that you become a vegan because you are hungry to have something to be about, something to be for, something to be against. In my collegiate era the Vietnam War, not food, galvanized us. You were for it or, as my friends and I were, passionately against it.

Veganism, in my household, seems "against" me. I'm an unabashed omnivore. I love to eat new foods and to cook them. I still buy new cookbooks, most recently (perhaps in an unconscious fit of anti-veganism) one called *A Passion for Cheese.* I'm in favor of expanding, not contracting, my palate. And I like nothing better than cooking new dishes for family and friends. Of necessity, I've learned to cook vegan meals, but it's a joyless endeavor. Veganism is about denial, about doing without. It's an uninspiring, barren "cuisine."

Thanksgiving night I watched my daughter and her friend pull, then eat the chewy Tofurkey "wishsticks." As a non-participant, I wasn't entitled to a wish, but I made one anyway. I wished fervently that she would eat meat again, or at the very least cheese and milk and eggs. She's going to Italy next year to spend her junior year in college abroad. How can she be a vegan and live amicably with a family in Tuscany for part of that time? Food is the gateway to other cultures, and eating a culture's food is one of the most basic acts of friendship. A cultural ambassador can't refuse the food. To her credit she realizes this and said that before she goes she will try and eat eggs, cheese and milk once a week so that she can eat her hosts' food without getting sick. Without getting sick! Is it so onerous, so foreign, to eat these things she was raised on, these things that are in her very bones?

When my daughter was a toddler, I marveled that she loved everything edible. She eagerly tried new foods, including raw mushrooms, smoked fish, and *escargot.* And she liked them all. But I remember well the first time she turned down the sustenance I offered. She was nearly two and still nursing when one evening her father suggested she might want watermelon instead of "hungry-time," as she had come to call breast-feeding. "Oh boy, watermelon," she enthused. And with that, she, but not I, was weaned.

The Tofurkey snapshot makes a great refrigerator photo, and not just because it's about food. I like it because my daughter looks genuinely happy and healthy and totally pleased with this odd food that hasn't come from my kitchen. Inadvertently I place the photo beside one of me taken last May. I'm sitting on the Alaskan tundra with my meat-eating Nunamiut friend, plucking a Canadian goose, and I'm smiling just as hard as my daughter.

There on the fridge we remain, birds in hand, 3500 miles − and worlds − apart.

COMPLAINT

BY LYNNE MARTIN BOWMAN

I eat and it does not please me –
the apple, the pear, the sweet ice cream,
the lettuce, the steak, the buttered potato –
no food fills, no tea soothes,
the pot boils, the kettle whistles emergency,
but I don't run to the fire.

Outside the sky burns clear blue
and the trees rise up to hold it,
budding red and pink and green
like hope without hands, without words,
with only water, light and air for food,
stuck in the ground, simply alive –

I raise my hands in the sun –
this way I will plant myself in the sky,
let my toes go to roots, let my hair
fly in the wind, maybe there find a new way
of eating, plate clean, the pattern evident.

THE GOLDEN APPLE

BY ALYSSA BRODY

n six months, everything will have changed. In six months, the fraternity boys, the transvestites, the homeless guys, the junkies, the jocks and everyone else who always hangs around will be drinking their beers, sipping their coffee, smoking their cigarettes, and eating their pizza somewhere else. In six months, all of this will have disappeared.

Today, I roll out of bed as usual 15 minutes before I'm supposed to be there and make my way down the windy street yawning and shivering. When I walk in the door, there is one customer sitting in a back booth eating his greasy breakfast. Arturo is cleaning the front windows and The Golden Apple sign with Windex and a dirty rag. He speaks virtually no English, so I just give him a wave. All of the Mexicans at The Apple work a full eight or nine hours there and also have jobs at other restaurants.

In the back, I gallantly offer to prep the salad bar because Sarah never washes the vegetables. My gesture seems futile, however, when I remember that Timothy is the head cook today. There are lots of alleged dirty secrets at The Apple, but when I hear that Timothy's a crackhead, I have to say it's not a bad guess. Whatever drugs he does have not helped his personality any, nor his appearance, nor his hygiene; it is barely 9:30 and he is already yelling at Barb for something or other, spit flying out through holes where teeth should have been. "You're such an asshole," she yells back. This is commonplace. Nobody so much as raises an eyebrow, including Fred, the owner, who has other worries on his mind.

His son, Tommy, has supposedly taken over the restaurant, but rumor has it that he is totally irresponsible and is squandering all kinds of money on cocaine. Even at such a crazy place, this sounds awfully dramatic to me, but it sure seems true. Tommy is always running around on fast-forward, and his eyes look especially buggy after he resurfaces from his office in the basement, which is off limits to us. One time I went to a party at some Apple guy's house, where it was all high school and college kids hanging out, and there was Tommy, drunk as a freshman girl at a frat party. This was at two in the morning on a Thursday night, and I couldn't help but wonder where his wife and kids thought he was as he smoked a joint with two pizza cooks and a cocktail waitress. Anyway, Fred is a pretty old guy, and it is sad to see him all stressed out and working so hard all of the time. Barb is the one who is always pointing it out, because she has been working here for over 20 years and knows everything that goes on at the place. I can hear her muttering under her breath about Tommy being a scumbag as she refills the saltshakers.

I go out to the front and my section is starting to fill up with the hangover crew. It is Saturday morning and the college kids shuffle in and order coffee as they light their first cigarettes of the day. It is a game day, and I can already tell that it is going to be hell. Every home game, these out-of-towners come in to eat breakfast before they go down to the stadium, and it gets so busy that even if they come three hours early, we manage to make them late for the game. We are all so unorganized that it gets backed up right away as soon as it gets crowded. The cooks start missing orders and we waitresses are so swamped that we forget to punch half of them in. Sure enough, the lady at table 24 is pissed because her toast came after she was already done eating, and another guy's mad because his omelet was cold and I couldn't bring him his bacon because every time the cook would put an order up in the window, another waitress would take it for her table. Sarah is yelling at Barb and Barb is yelling at me and we are all yelling at Timothy and Fred is yelling at all of us. The customers are yelling at the waitresses and the manager is yelling at the customers. Then Tommy yells at the manager. Finally the out-of-towners all leave, never to come again, and we are happy to be left with the locals and the college students.

Everyone is ordering pizzas and beer now, so life is much easier. The Golden Apple is famous for its pizza. I go into the back room to sneak a cigarette and talk with Rico while he is making dough. "Hey, *Mamacita*," he says. I ask him why Barb is crying. She cries at least once a day, and whatever is wrong is usually something so strange and horrible that you don't know what to say. "Kevin is missing again," Rico says, rolling up his sleeves and pouring beer into the dense batter. Kevin is Barb's boyfriend. He has a habit of taking the truck and disappearing for weeks, whatever that means. And Barb is distraught the whole time because she doesn't know where he is and she is worried and he took all of their money, and she says she hates him. Then he eventually comes back and everything is fine until it starts all over again. Sarah covers my tables and I run home to bring Barb a Popsicle from my freezer, because she loves them. When I give it to her, she starts crying again. If you're too nice to her, she always cries.

Meanwhile, Miss Melissa has arrived. She makes a scene as always, pushing her way through the kitchen on her way to the back to make pizzas. She is about six foot four and weighs around 300 pounds. She has long, curly black hair with lots of Soul Glo on it and spiky fake nails that are pink today, with gold glitter. Oh yes, and she's really a man. She gives my butt a little pinch as she walks by. "Look at yo little Pippy Longstockin' shit! Them braids is just so precious, Girlfriend. What ch'yall doin tonight, sweetheart? Come see Miss Melissa in action." She hands me a flyer for her evening performance and breezes past me.

"I've seen it," says Sarah. "Don't go." Before I can answer, Francisco shows up. He makes pizzas, too, and he is also about 300 pounds. He, however, has a moustache.

"You ladies wanna smoke some weed?" We warn him that Mama is around, but he shrugs and slips into the back alley. Mama is Fred's mother and Tommy's grandmother. She is old as hell and long since retired, but when she lumbers in from her apartment upstairs, she is the boss. Everyone bends over backwards to kiss her ass, and it isn't easy to keep her happy.

Up front, the game is in full swing. Michigan is ahead by three, and everyone is getting wasted. Tommy's cousin Tina is bartending, but it is so busy that Sarah and I are pouring drinks, too. When Tina's back is turned, we fill up our Cokes with rum and Jack Daniels respectively. Barb never drinks at work. She waits until five and then doesn't stop until she passes out. She is thin as a sheet of paper and eats practically nothing, but drinks like a Russian soldier.

I have a table of rowdy jocks in the back of the restaurant, and they have already consumed about four pizzas, eight pitchers and a thousand chicken wings. I bring them another pitcher but I notice that one guy is not looking so hot. I cut him off, and he starts to make a scene. After Francisco throws him out, Tommy reprimands me for letting the guy get so drunk. It's hard to take him seriously, however, when his darting eyes are practically bulging out of his head, probably from all the blow he's been snorting in the basement. Finally, the game ends, and all of the drunks begin to scatter noisily, happy or belligerent, depending on who they rooted for. It is early afternoon, and quiet again. A pretty girl and a guy from the basketball team are slurping milkshakes. There are four construction workers drinking beer and eating hamburgers in the front. An older lady is drinking lemonade and drawing with pastels. Three guys with piercings all over their faces and tattoos everywhere sit down and cheerily order a pizza. Gabe, one of the cooks, is hunched in the corner doing math problems. He's a mathematics genius. He thinks formulas and calculations are beautiful, and that there is a mathematical explanation for everything. I got a C in Calculus, so I just take his word for it.

The regulars who have been avoiding the football crowd lurk in and reclaim their places as Rico replaces an empty keg behind the bar. There is Mr. Wernick, the guy in the bright orange hat who never talks, and there is the guy with the fuzzy white hair and beard who orders coffee and rice pudding. Jerry-from-Brooklyn arrives in a good mood, and before he settles in with his first bottle of white zinfandel, he gives us $10 for the jukebox and lets us pick the songs. My friend Mike comes in to visit and orders chili and French toast because he cannot decide between them. I try to stealthily smoke a cigarette that is resting in an ashtray on the edge of his table, but it's more trouble than it's worth, so I go with Barb to the bathroom. That is the rule: Unless you are on your one official break of the day, you have to go into the bathroom and lock the door if you want to smoke. Mama gets mad if you smoke in front of the customers, and you never know when she'll show up.

Now she sits her huge body in the back corner, and we all rush to put cushions on her chair and bring her coffee. "Oh, Honey," she cries in her thick Greek accent, "Oh, Honey, thank you. It's so hard, you know. Oh, Honey!" Two of the cooks are resting in the front room while there are no orders in, and she starts shrieking and yelling at them in Greek. They yell back at first, but Fred pushes them into the kitchen. Mama sits back down and pats my hand. "Oh, Honey! You the *best*. I tell Tommy." Last week she tried to fire me because I didn't refill some guy's water glass soon enough.

At five the early evening crowd starts to trickle in. I notice that the scary transsexual is in Sarah's section. I feel bad for her, but I can't help but feel relieved for me. He/She/It always wears a musty old white dress that is yellowing from age, a strand of fake pearls, and tons of makeup, especially rouge. Today he/she/it has on red pumps and chipping red nail polish. Staring blankly ahead, every move is slow and eerie. Eyelids inevitably begin to droop as a pale hand slowly lifts a cigarette to smeary red lips or smooths some stringy long hair. He/She/It never speaks except to order coffee, but sits there nodding and smoking away and freaking everyone out for hours.

While I count out my tip money and put some aside for the bartender, Barb asks me if I want to go next door to Harley's for a drink. She is sitting on the flour sacks in the back of the kitchen, her skinny legs dangling like a child's. It is a funny sight, especially because her face looks so old, and her hair is thinning and streaked with gray. She is only 40, but looks 20 years older. It's painful to contemplate the depths of her problems. Some days I can put them in the back of my mind, but now I am disturbed. I shudder. "I can't today," I say, thinking that there will be infinite tomorrows to make it up to her.

But I'm wrong. In two months, I will quit. In four months, I will move away. In six months, this will all disappear. The restaurant will go under. For the first time in almost 40 years, The Golden Apple will open with new owners. The restaurant will be bright and clean. The waitresses will wear blue polo shirts and khaki pants. Average looking people will eat pasta and dinner salads and "Mama's Spinach Pie" while watching *Jeopardy* on the big screen TV over the brand new bar. When I walk down the familiar Ann Arbor streets expecting to see the old place, expecting to see Tommy and his buggy eyes, expecting to see Barb and apologize for not keeping in touch, I will see instead a bunch of strangers. A few of the old photos will remain, matted in brand new, shiny silver frames.

On the wall, I will see Barb. In that picture, she is 20 years old. It is the 1979 Ann Arbor Art Fair, and she stands on the crowded sidewalk in her apron, next to two other waitresses who have long since become lawyers or cosmetologists or teachers. Her hair is long. Her face looks young, but she looks uncomfortable somehow, as if she doesn't want proof of her life's path in a photograph.

As I walk through the kitchen, people I don't recognize will stare at me as they cut up vegetables. "Hey, *Mamacita.*" The familiar voice will fill me with relief. Rico and I will hug and go in the back to talk. "Tommy, he lose the place," he will tell me, handing me a lump of pizza dough to play with. "Almost everybody fired."

"And Barb," I'll ask.

"She fired, too. She live now in New Orleans, with Kevin." I will try to sense an aura of the old place in the air, and it will dawn on me that consistency is the anomaly, not change.

I will think of her picture on the wall and try to envision Barb in another town, with another life. It will be as difficult for me to imagine as it must have been for her. When I ask Rico if she's happy, he will shrug, poking a finger into the center of the dough. "What do you think?"

JELL-O GIRL

BY LISA BROSNAN

irst days at work tend to confuse. This didn't disturb me when I started my job at the casino boat because, as a cocktail waitress, this is pretty much my usual state anyway. But I would go so far as to say I was misled here – bamboozled, even. Please remember that this is a place where even the carpeting is designed to perplex and disorientate. Before I was allowed out on the floor, my manager, we'll call him Derf, made clear to me three very important things about the casino where I work. He told me that our casino was not a gambling business, but an entertainment experience. He told me that our entertainment experience was better than all other entertainment experiences because of the quality of our customer service, provided by our family of employees, whom he referred to as "our greatest asset." He told me that this family of employees is well taken care of by the casino, which he referred to as "a wonderful place to work." He also said that my uniform would be provided, as if I had thought I'd actually have to go out and buy something so tacky. And he told me that the casino would furnish all my meals free of charge. This, he called a benefit.

Some folks get paid sick leave and personal days. Some folks get 401K plans run by competent financial advisors. Some are even vested in less than 10 years. We get free meals. I told Derf I wanted in.

At the casino where I work, benefits are not to be confused with bonuses. A bonus happens on special occasions. Benefits are taken for granted throughout the year. Every year, each employee is given a ham for Christmas. This is an example of a bonus – our Christmas bonus in its entirety. This bonus ham is given to employees of seven years as well as to employees of seven days. Even the vegetarians are entitled to their Christmas ham. I call this "The Great Ham Giveaway." I know, I should be grateful and I am. But I am also suspicious. You see, there is a reason why the casino takes the trouble to provide us with actual, physical hams for the holiday rather than simply enclosing a gift certificate for a ham in our annual Christmas card. Someone got a damn good deal on those hams. It is entirely possible that they fell off a truck. Yes, in the past, we have been given out-of-date hams. These old hams had a slight greenish hue to them. So every year, I politely pass on my Christmas bonus. Green, however festive, is not a color I want for my ham.

Hams unclaimed by the employees of the casino where I work are donated to charity. The casino's publicity department makes note of this every chance it gets as a demonstration of how the casino is a generous and benevolent place for the community as well as for the employees. I am sure it is only a coincidence that for several weeks after "The Great Ham Giveaway" some form of ham is present in nearly every dish at the employee cafeteria. I suspect that these hams have been detoured to our break room by Derf who, if pressed, would swear up and down that he really doesn't know how they got there.

Besides ham, the employee cafeteria offers a wide ranging variety of exotic foods including: creamed chicken, creamed corn, Cream of Wheat, and salad greens that look suspiciously fresh. Soup is either white or brown or, sometimes, green. I stay away from the white soup because it is rumored to be made with Cremora rather than cream and because it has a tendency to cause widespread gastronomic distress. Brown soup is usually okay if it isn't too cloudy and if all of the chunks have a clear and identifiable purpose. No one knows what's in the green soup. All manner of scrumptious cakes, pies, and cookies can be found throughout the day in the dessert case. At least, they may have been scrumptious before they were picked over by our customers at the buffet. I call these treats "The desserts not chosen" – and I stay away from them.

Of all the foods that come and go through the employee cafeteria, there is one mainstay, something that can always be counted on. This is the green Jell-O. The reason it is always there on the top shelf of the dessert case is because no one eats it. It sits poised like a pit boss over the shoulder of a rookie dealer. It just sits there, waiting, in little plastic cups. I must admit that I never paid much attention to it. That is, until that fateful day when I entered the employee break room in search of a mid-afternoon snack. What happened between me and the green Jell-O is still too difficult to relate. The pain of the experience will haunt me as long as I can feel the dent it left at the top of my head, so I am including an account of this occurrence exactly as it appeared in the official casino employee incident report.

Minding my own business, I went to the employee break room to acquire fruit for my mid-afternoon smoothie. As I slid the door to the desert case open and reached for a particularly ripe orange, a rogue green Jell-O jumped out and hit me over the head. I was beaned. Now, I had always thought of Jell-O as a rather benign dessert item. I may have gotten this impression from the song, "They call it mellow Jell-O..." The other Jell-Os in the case have always been very well mannered. I've never had a problem with the red or even the yellow Jell-O.

I hold Food and Beverage Manager Derf personally liable for this incident as he is ultimately responsible for the actions of all gelatinous desserts on the boat. Marine Manager Puddley is also at fault for not having the appropriate warning signs posted. There should be a sign: "Caution – Falling Desserts" or "Beware The Green Jell-O." A little yellow caution tape around the dessert case wouldn't hurt, either.

This incident has been very traumatic for me and my family. I am now afraid to enter the employee break room, afraid to eat green food, and I get all shaky when I see Bill Cosby on TV. I am terrified beyond belief to even be in the same room with green Jell-O.

Needless to say, this has greatly affected my sex life.

Please, please, please remove the green Jell-O from the employee break room and all of its fellow Jell-Os: red, yellow, and orange (just in case) before this happens to someone else.

There is a space on the incident report form to list any witnesses to the event. I had numerous witnesses to this episode, but I couldn't make out who they were because their faces were so contorted with laughter. Apparently, some of my fellow employees, employees I am to consider as family, see great humor in other people's misfortunes.

I have submitted this report to the heads of security, surveillance, food and beverage, and marine operations, as well as to the general manager of the casino itself. To date, nothing at all has been done about the green Jell-O. It still sits, lurking, at the top of the dessert case. Unassuming employees still pass by the dessert case unaware of the dangers within. The only difference now is that the general manager calls me Jell-O Girl when he passes through my section.

All goes to show that things are not always what they seem. An entertainment experience could, after all, be only gambling. A Christmas bonus could turn out to be a green ham. And an employee benefit may prove a hazardous dessert.

IF I WERE YOUR TUMS

BY LINDA BROWN

I would be pastel –
the melt in your mouth
kind –
pretty and smooth ,
and perfectly round
like your other women,
the ones I'm not
supposed to know about.

You would reach for me
after dinner
and I would lodge
in your intestines
somewhere between
your gall and your guile,
your grating voice and
ingratiating ways,
offering as much relief
as you have given me
with your false elixir,
love.

LESSONS FROM A FOOD THIEF

BY UTE CARSON

W e had arrived in the West after fleeing from the Russian troops – safe. Spring oozed in as warm as a lagoon, with trees just leafing out and meadows starred with anemones. The Second World War was nearly over. But the post-war chaos was about to begin.

My father had been killed at the beginning of the war. Two years later, pregnant with my sister Anne, my mother remarried. Her second husband was a Count who had spent his youth on the battlefront. On leave, he searched for a mate and found my mother, but he was not prepared for a pregnancy and even less for me, a vivacious five-year-old.

"I need my freedom, not more obligations," he shouted at my mother when she gave him the news of her pregnancy.

But the Count had been raised in a family where the code of *noblesse oblige* still held sway, so when the war ended, he dutifully married my mother and adopted me.

The nobleman and I were thrown together by necessity.

"Come on, you little shit," he told me, "If I'm going to have to put up with you, you'll have to help me make ends meet."

And that's why I began to steal.

I became a thief, a lavish thief, a food thief. My stepfather was my instructor and I, his eager pupil. I was by then no longer a toddler but a little girl of six.　◇◇◇

It started with raids on coal trains. On the outskirts of our town, the loud-squeaking trains had to slow down and were often halted completely by a red and white signal before moving on to a single track leading into the train station. Whenever a coal train stopped, the word spread like wildfire from house to house: "Coal train – coal train." The Count would sprint away and I'd be right behind him, armed with several burlap sacks. He had already jumped on a train car by the time I arrived, wishing for grasshopper legs so I wouldn't lag behind.

The Count threw coal down in my direction, using his hands like huge shovels. I gathered the chunks as fast as I could and filled the bags. Together we dragged the coal home and hid it behind bushes in our garden where I stood guard until nightfall when the Count would empty our loot down the coal chute into the cellar. Once in a while a policeman caught us and confiscated the coal.

"He'll keep every bit of it for himself," the Count grumbled. "You can't tell me he hands it over to the authorities."

The Allies were the new authorities and they were baffled by our strange wheeling and dealing. Without coal we could not keep warm, and there would be no fire for preparing what we needed most, food.

Mint tea leaves which once grew abundantly along streams or brooks became a rare commodity we traded. Wearing old winter gloves, we also harvested nettles and boiled the leaves to make soup. We were experts in gathering edible mushrooms from cow dung and from the soft moss along the forest floor. I learned to distinguish nonpoisonous from poisonous ones by color, shape, the texture of their lamella and by an acid, foul or sweet-sour smell. I also became skilled at plundering elderberry bushes, reaching for a low branch and pulling it down to my level. I would then scoop the white blossoms into my basket and later my mother boiled them into a delicious, sugary brew. From the elderberries themselves we squeezed an ink-blue juice. Everything was used. In the fall acorns were cracked open and the soft contents eaten or pressed into cooking oil. After the wheat had been brought in from the fields, women gathered fallen husks into their aprons and later shucked and ground them into flour. Even carrots we sometimes gleaned. And if they were a little rotten, I smuggled them away for my pet rabbit, Flopsy.

But the natural harvest was limited and the sites of these foods were soon swarming with people quarreling over the diminishing supply.

So we stole.

◇ ◇ ◇

Private fields and gardens were our first forbidden targets. I did my best there. I climbed on fence posts where I could survey the terrain, then give an "all clear" to the Count. Sometimes we stuffed our mouths so full we had chipmunk cheeks as we plundered a raspberry bush or pilfered strawberries from a patch.

This is when I learned to whistle through my fingers and I learned to fight.

My basket was filled with pears one day when a boy, pretending to amble by, reached over and dumped the basket. He started grabbing handfuls of my fruit right in front of me. I whistled sharply for help.

The Count was already watching. "Don't let him do that."

"Stay out of my way," the boy snarled.

Suddenly I lunged at him and shoved him back. He reached for my sweater, the one my mother had knitted from leftover yarn, and I saw it begin to unravel. I pulled back; he tore more sweater. So I punched him hard in the nose. He put his hand up as a guard over his bloody nose, left the pears behind and ran.

◇ ◇ ◇

During the post-war era farmers fared best because they raised their own produce and also kept poultry as well as livestock. When we heard that a pig had been butchered, we took an heirloom or a piece of jewelry to trade for some liver, a kidney, or that rare delicacy, bits of the brain. My mother fried them with scrambled eggs.

A dead pig was strung up by its hind feet in the open entrance of a barn, then sliced down the middle and swung back like the sides of a door. The blood was gathered in a pail, vital organs were carefully removed, and chunks of meat tenderly carved from the body, each slice worth its weight in gold.

I hated the sight of a slaughtered pig and usually squinted up into the clouds where I imagined it alive and well. Some clouds were puffed up like feathers, others stretched along the horizon like elephant trunks, others resembled the forelocks of sheep.

One night the Count and I sneaked up to a pig which had been butchered that evening, cleaned and stripped, the carcass hanging out to dry with flies taking their share of the leftover meat. With one deft stroke the Count cut two long slivers from a thigh and stuffed them into the front of his shirt. He wiped the blade of his pocket knife, snapped it shut and we ambled home, nonchalant.

◇ ◇ ◇

There were no colorful outdoor markets after the war. But the black market flourished, especially with food. My sister Anne was born late that fall and my mother pumped extra milk. I remember tears dripping from her eyes onto little Anne's face as the baby

—◈— 47 —◈—

sucked on cracked and swollen breasts. My mother stimulated her milk production by nursing Anne for awhile and then pumping extra milk. Often baby Anne was put back into her crib hungry. She only whimpered though, having adjusted to post-war scarcity like the rest of us.

The Count and I made daily trips around town to sell the precious ounces. He found his customers, often women short on milk for their own babies. Many of the women lacked attention as well, and I became a witness to the Count's frequent stopovers. I was told to wait in a foyer among umbrellas in metal stands and winter coats reeking of moisture and stale sweat, or in a warm kitchen where I slumped into a chair, dozing after our long outings. Sometimes a dog or a cat would streak by my leg, and I got to play for a while. When the Count reemerged, I was often given a treat by the women, a peach, fuzzy as little Anne's head or a slice of freshly baked bread smelling of yeast.

"Now, don't tell your mother about our stops," the Count warned me. "It might upset her."

I was confused but decided to keep these secret visits to myself since my mother was so sad all the time as it was.

◇ ◇ ◇

In the broken down shed behind our house the Count kept his prize possession, a rusty, rattling woman's bicycle with crooked handlebars and no lights. Bakeries began to operate again before most other shops reopened. And as before the war, shopkeepers set out their baked goods, the stuff of life, in large baskets first thing in the morning. I straddled the bent handlebars as the Count pedaled us to a bakery around the corner. There I slipped down and bolted past the store quick as a weasel, grabbing a roll or two without missing a step. At the end of the street he would swing me back onto the handlebars, his right arm hooked under one of my armpits. Because the shop owners were quick to shout for the police and ready to chase me with a broom, we pulled this trick on only a few occasions.

On the other hand, like the fox in the fairy tale, we continually raided chicken coops for eggs, and when we felt extra lucky, we would catch a squawking hen or duck. While I looked away, the Count would twist the fowl's neck. A catch like that would fill our cooking pot for weeks. After the meat and skin had been consumed, my mother boiled the bones, extracting rich nourishment from the marrow.

I saw my first black man, an American soldier, in a chicken coop. He was gathering eggs in his helmet. He offered me chewing gum which I was afraid to touch, not knowing what it was. The Count said it was safe to take, so I grabbed the gift and stuffed it into my pocket.

◇ ◇ ◇

We invited friends and neighbors to a special Christmas meal. On the table decorated with fir branches, pine cones and candles stood a steaming roast, spiced with thyme and caraway seeds. Before we sat down, I rushed outside to feed my Flopsy rabbit, the one I had raised on spinach leaves and stolen carrots. The hutch was empty. I knew immediately that the "duck" my mother had so lovingly prepared was no duck at all but my pet rabbit. I said nothing as I plopped down next to our neighbor, Mr. Martin, who was asked to say grace and complied with a long, heartfelt prayer, his crippled, arthritic fingers laced together. But I burst into tears when the Count started carving. Then my mother said she couldn't eat. I felt the Count's eyes on me. After a few bites, he too pushed his plate away. Was this thieving stranger becoming my father?

Our guests filled their stomachs until they could eat no more, then held their sides with clammy palms and let off satisfied puffing sounds, like steam escaping from the engine of a coal freighter.

◇ ◇ ◇

Once we were caught stealing sugar-beets. Boiled beets, stirred into molasses, made a spread as tasty as jam or honey. That evening a policeman surprised us just as my stepfather was saying, "Let's quit. We have enough."

The Count could talk himself out of any situation but that evening, his clever tongue deserted him and we were booked. The Count's face turned lobster-red with embarrassment as he stumbled over his words,

"Officer − it won't happen again − please." But we had been warned before.

The night in jail was a humiliation for Nobleman Count Friederich and an adventure for me. I had been parted from my family before when I was hospitalized for several weeks, so I took the separation lightly. I was taken to a cell where four women were curled up on bare mattresses. They got up and fussed over me and gave me their only blanket. The jailers served us split pea soup that we slurped with relish, watery broth with floury lumps swimming on the surface.

"Get that damn mouse," a woman squealed while on the way to the toilet pail. She had slipped on the furry paw as the tiny thing had headed for her shoes.

I tried to catch the soft gray creature, but had no luck. How could anyone make such a racket over a little mouse? I had once spotted a rat as big as a cat carrying off one of little Anne's baby socks.

Count Friederich and I were released the next morning without breakfast. The Count seemed glad to see me and put his hand on my shoulder as we walked away together.

When we arrived back home, my mother was inconsolable. "I just knew something terrible had happened to you."

I waited until she calmed down to tell her about the marvelous soup.

◇ ◇ ◇

Having once experienced food as a scarcity, I know few boundaries. "Please help yourself," is my attitude.

In my childhood food separated the satiated from the hungry. Christmas dinner was a communion even if the roast was my rabbit. And food served as a bond between two thieves, a Count and his little accomplice.

But I am frugal to the point of stinginess. My lean years as a youthful thief are long over but not forgotten. My present plenitude has made me want to share, even though I realize that I can't feed all the starving people of the world. But also, in small measure, I do what I can never to be wasteful. I scowl if my dinner guests leave a morsel on their plates. I take along plastic containers whenever we dine out, be it at McDonald's or the Ritz. I eat moldy bread, week-old leftovers, and seldom throw away a scrap. My family wonders why I have never gotten food poisoning.

◇ ◇ ◇

Once a thief, always a thief.

I gladly gave up my thieving for being a paying customer at Kroger and Safeway. But I never acquired the conviction that stealing is wrong. I know we can't live together without respecting each other's property, and I do enjoy my material possessions and want to protect them. Still, I never developed a moral stance against stealing. Even when I look at a picture in an art exhibit and consider buying it, my first impulse is simply to take it. I especially have trouble passing my neighbor's flower garden when the vases at my house are empty and his roses are in bloom. I have learned to ask, but I would have no qualms about just picking one or two without his permission.

Two years ago my childhood bicycle was stolen, an antique with a "Bismarck" insignia. When the police recovered it and asked me if I wanted the thief booked, I replied, "No, I've been there. Just help me straighten the spokes."

CHOCOLATE BAR

BY MAUREEN CONNOLLY

What we need
Is a Chocolate Bar
A Grateful Dead-esque kind of place
To sit melted together
With women and men
Eating eclairs
And knocking back gin.
Or licking and flicking
Fine chocolate *mousse*
Followed by chasers
Of full-proof vermouth.
White chocolate pieces
Like cream from the breast
Riding the lips
And warming the chest.
Balls of milk chocolate
Smoothness along
The soft inside mouth
And the back of the tongue.
But, oh! that dark chocolate
It makes you talk a lot
Leading to dreams
Of the richest ice creams.
Endorphins are rising
It's so energizing
We're sipping on mocha
We may start to polka...
In the sweet late late night
Women and men
Sitting in trances
Slide into Godiva
And chocolate romances.

CONFESSIONS OF THE OMELET KING
BY GREG COOK

et me tell you a true story: I could cook up to 16 omelets at a time when I was a cook in the Navy. Granted, my trusty sidekick Fred took the orders for me. I was obscenely young (18) at the time, and we were in the Indian Ocean for a good cause (to free the hostages in Iran), but I still think it stands as a pretty good accomplishment. For a few weeks, I was the omelet king of the aircraft carrier *Coral Sea*, and I wore that crown with pride and distinction. Kings, however, come and go, and I lost the crown for several reasons. In particular, there was one petty officer who dogged me my whole time on board, and he as much as anyone helped cast me from the ranks of royalty.

Before going aboard *Coral Sea* I went to Boot Camp and then cooking school. Because I had enjoyed a high school cooking class, I decided to try cooking for Uncle Sam. Of course the military could not simply call us cooks; we were designated "Mess Management Specialists." The class rolled out of barracks early – before dawn – to learn cooking in large quantities. We practiced using military menus which were calculated based on servings for 100. Preparing the dish then became a matter of math: to serve 765 people, we'd multiply the ingredients by 7.65. We gained familiarity with the basic cooking tools: fryers, ovens, coppers (large cauldrons), steamers and grills. We sat through classes on baking, nutrition, and sanitation and repeated and practiced our mantra: "clean as you go."

Clean as you go – that's one valuable thing I learned there. If there are a few minutes while something is cooking, take that time to set aside dirty utensils, wipe down surfaces, or sweep and mop. There was much more to learn about cleaning and sanitation, such as the proper temperatures for storing food and sanitizing utensils, and the need to rotate supplies. We returned from classes wet, our uniforms and skin covered with flour or other ingredients, and smelling like pot roast, pepper steak, fried rice or whatever we'd cooked that day. But I made it through school with no inkling of what lay ahead for me in the *Coral Sea's* kitchens.

The ship was docked at Subic Bay Naval Base, preparing to sail out to the Indian Ocean. I stood before the 1,000 foot gray hulk, sea bag on my back and uniform hat on my head, wearing a black wool outfit known as the "monkey suit" and feeling like anything but a king. My first assignment kept me out of the galleys (kitchens). I was part of a crew which gathered supplies from storage compartments on various parts of the ship, shivered in the meat freezers and vegetable compartments, and sweated in the confined rooms below decks where the canned goods lay. We brought those items back to the various kitchens and bakeries. I began to observe the military system in action and the adversarial hierarchy in charge of my division. And I got to meet my nemesis.

His name was Petty Officer First Class Reasonable. He was a Filipino, and so the correct pronunciation of his name was RAY-SUN-AH-BLAY, but of course everyone called him Reasonable. No one I have ever known has been more inappropriately named. He looked like an Asian Churchill, stocky, scowling, face like a bulldog. He barked like a bulldog too, and I still shudder when I think of him howling my name above the rattling cauldrons and crackling deep fryers in the Coral Sea's main galley as perspiration rolled off his brown face. I wanted to go jump overboard because of my failures.

I truly got to know Reasonable during my time in that galley. I was rotated in there after a few weeks on the supply crew and a bout of mononucleosis which kept me out of action for nearly a week. I wasn't an apt pupil in the busy breakfast shift: sweating and cursing, I broke yoke after yoke on the grill, cooking eggs to order. People complained that the over-easy were too runny, or the over-hard were undercooked. The heat from the grill, noise of clanging pots, and standing in one spot for several hours made me wonder why I'd listened to my recruiter back home.

Lunch was no better. I was clumsy opening cans and had no flair for ordinary dishes like soup. The bosses didn't trust me with the ovens, and I seemed to get in everybody's way around the steamers and fryers. For whatever reason, they did not send me to the "Doggie Diner," the Coral Sea's version of fast food cookery. Instead I stayed under Reasonable's critical glowering.

But then, somehow, I started to shine as the omelet cook. I cracked hundreds of eggs by hand at night with great dexterity, breaking one in each hand by tapping it on the edge of a huge pot, then deftly opening the shells wide with just my fingers as the contents fell into the mixture below. As supplies of fresh eggs grew scarce, I thawed cartons of frozen eggs. With my assistant Fred, I devised a system for taking orders and keeping the different requests straight. I varied the temperature on parts of the grill and laid out my ingredients – onions, peppers, mushrooms, ham, cheese – based on typical numbers of requests. Ham and cheese was the most popular choice. I scooped the large ladle in and out of the egg container with speed, setting down in quick succession 16 golden yellow circles of beaten egg to begin sizzling into omelets. My line moved with speed and efficiency, and my fellow sailors recognized me as "Cookie," the one who made their omelets.

Word spread, and more men came through my line. I was a mini-celebrity onboard the *Coral Sea*. Reasonable had no complaints, though he or one of his colleagues would scrutinize my grill and work area during inspection. Usually, that clean-as-you-go training kept me immune, though occasionally I would be forced to spend valuable time (we worked daily 12-hour shifts) cleaning the grill and the area around it before I could leave for my living quarters.

As the cruise wore on, our supplies of fresh food diminished: homogenized milk gave way to canned and sterilized or ultra-pasteurized in little individual boxes from Singapore. The lettuce rotted, and we ran out of our fresh fruits and vegetables. We also ran out of all eggs except in powdered form, and powdered eggs won't work for omelets. My reign came to an end, and Reasonable found new joy in hovering over my inept attempts at steaming vegetables or frying fish.

I was reassigned to the aft bake shop, and so for a while I escaped the relentless criticism of my culinary nemesis. Our mission in the bake shop was simple: turn out enough donuts, cinnamon rolls and coffee cake every day for breakfast and make some pies and cakes as well. Our biggest task each night was to carve up a tremendous mound of dough into donuts and then fry them; or roll it out by hand into long cinnamon and sugar-filled tubes, then use a rectangular wooden-handled dough knife to cut them into individual rolls laid out on sheet pans. We worked out an assembly line for making the donuts, with someone placing the puffy dough into the six-foot-long metal fryer and another snatching them out with tongs, like Scylla plucking Odysseus' men out of the sea. Another member of our crew would roll them in sugar or coat them with glaze made from confectioner's sugar. I gained quite a few pounds during my stint there.

The warm, sugary pastry smell always drew a few hungry-looking sailors to our door, and we learned that food could be a valuable commodity in our ship's economy. Still-warm donuts or gooey cinnamon rolls bought clothing, drugs, or even information and favors. Coffee cake, even with sweet streusel topping and loaded with blueberries, did not buy much.

Making cakes was problematic – we had to cope with one of the ship's idiosyncrasies, the permanent tilt (the result of an angled flight deck added on after initial construction), which led to our cakes being thicker at one end. I was no longer the king, but my colleagues and I at the bake shop had a nice little gig. Because we worked at night, there was little scrutiny of our activities. It also meant Reasonable rarely came around.

After a few months I was reassigned, and I could not escape Reasonable and his cronies anymore. My request for a transfer and leave were denied, so after we returned to our home port of Alameda (San Francisco Bay), I went UA (Unauthorized Absence), the Navy equivalent of AWOL. The Omelet King AKA the Duke of Donuts was on the run, hounded from his throne by his enemies. Thwarted by circumstances and feeling desperate, I deserted the kitchens for a trip home to northern New York state. After a month, I returned to *Coral Sea* and turned myself in.

Scientists tell us humans evolved over the millennia to maximize food use. We store fat for emergencies. On the other hand, in many religious and ascetic traditions, adherents deny themselves food in an attempt at purification – they fast. But the fast can also be imposed as a form of punishment. Food deprivation can be a powerful weapon for a government or parent. In 1980, the Uniform Code of Military Justice allowed commanders to discipline troops by placing them on three days of bread and water. I know this because it happened to me.

Captain Dunleavy had plenty of reasons to punish me. My transgressions included disobeying orders, unauthorized absence, and escaping from custody. I wanted out of the military and away from the clutches of the relentless Reasonable; the captain wanted to give a young sailor a chance to shape up. As part of my sentence, I sat in a cell for three days with nothing to eat but white, sliced bread and water to drink. It's amazing how being surrounded by nearly unlimited food makes one *blasé*, whereas once one loses access to food – even the most basic – eating occupies the mind to a ridiculous extent.

My exile from kingship was made more onerous by two facts: first, the men guarding me knew me and had frequented my omelet line many times; second, I had to walk by the mess decks and near the galley to go to sick bay for a check-up. All those food smells – milk, gravy, hot grease from fryers, even the mixed odors from the scullery – taunted me, setting off gurgles in my stomach.

I survived, and even shaped up for a while. I was temporarily assigned to another division working on the rehab of the ship, and thus I kept out of the kitchen and Reasonable's way for a while. Eventually though, I went back to the galley and was at his mercy. Once again my ineptness kept him constantly hovering over me. I received the dirty jobs of cleaning the ovens or other filthy areas. He kept me away from what I could do, and forced me to do what I could not do.

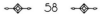 58

I remember one day in particular. I was assigned to cook pancakes on one of the grills. It seemed easy enough: make some batter by mixing together flour, water and other ingredients, cook some pancakes, put them in pans, and keep them warm until they were needed on the serving line. The menu called for pineapple pancakes, so I added a few cans of pineapple to the mixture. The batter tasted both sweet and tart, and the consistency seemed just right. Good pancake batter should spread out somewhat, but not be so thin it turns into a crepe once it is heated. As I went to turn them over on the grill, once the bubbles started to pop, something went wrong—a burning, charred smell rose up and they stuck and tore apart when I tried to slide the spatula underneath.

What the heck is going on? I wondered. *Maybe it's just the first batch as the grill gets adjusted,* I thought. But they continued to burn and stick and tear apart, reminding me about those lessons from school on presentation affecting taste. Before long, Reasonable was standing there, a disgusted look on his face, and I...I was close to crying right then. He yelled at me, "Cook!"

It turns out that pineapple, due to its enzymes and sugar content, needs to be drained and rinsed before being added to the batter.

Reasonable shook his head as I slumped my shoulders in defeat and shame, and he said, "Cook, you're pucked up." (In his language, Tagalog, "f" gets pronounced like "p.") Far from being a king, I was exiled from the kitchen, a failure.

The once-proud and accomplished Omelet King had lost his throne, and my enemy was triumphant. He'd shown me to be a loser, a peasant with no talent, unskilled. In the months after my discharge, I was a loser back home too, not the bake shop leader in charge of making donuts and desserts for several thousand hungry sailors. There have been times since then I've wished for a renewal of my innocence, my hubris, my faith – the faith which allowed me, *ME,* to cook 16 omelets and keep everyone happy. But now, at 40, I have a different perspective on it all.

No, I will never again be that boy who cooked 16 omelets, hoping for the release of the American hostages in Iran but also working on the perfect tan. The *Coral Sea* was de-commissioned years ago, replaced by a new, faster, larger and better-equipped carrier. It's enough that my taste buds and nose still work, that I keep on encountering new foods, and meeting new friends to eat with. It is enough that I was King, Omelet King, for that brief time. Let someone else pick up the crown, because I'm too busy tasting life.

JUST DESSERTS

BY MICHELE F. COOPER

She pares the apples with blue fire in her blade,
swipes the peels into the bag before the pile builds,
plunges the knife into white flesh, peels and peels.

She did the dough yesterday, pounded it into the
requisite ball, slamming it on the counter, each
thwack a drum roll and trumpet call. It doesn't

matter how sweet the cinnamon, how the dark brown
sugar softens her shaking hands and she watches it
fall between the apple pieces finding resting places

in the shadows waiting for heat and butter to start
raising a scent she can live with, 14 years of soap pads
and scouring powder having turned her to stone.

She likes the chemistry on her counter, the math of it,
6 or 7 Granny Smiths, 1/4 teaspoons of this and that,
sour cream dough she uses for everything,

sprinkles of nutmeg and allspice, handfuls of dark
sugar setting like hair on the round apple head.
When the big dots of butter melt, when the sugar

falls, the apples cook down, dough relaxes and
hardens and fragrantly browns, she'll have to stop
her confounded weeping at once, wipe her face

so she can take up the pan without tipping,
set it safely on the wooden board under the light
and decry the transformation that comes and goes

around the stove, thanks to her silver knife and
shakers. She wants to cook herself, wonders
how to undo her pupae to her caterpillar, her

caterpillar for her Monarch, there's a trick here
damn it, and it's not in her notebook where
she left it under Just Desserts.

CHEF'S FINEST

BY DONNA COUSINS

 hef stands inside the kitchen door peering through a window the size of a petri dish. His nose leaves a smudge on the glass. Beyond the door lies a long, succulent landscape of carved fruits and vegetables, marinated meats, fish and fowl paired with rich simmered sauces – a vast buffet stretching end-to-end across a gilded banquet hall to a distant horizon dense with sweets. In adjacent candle-lit reception rooms, champagne is working its salubrious ways on a hundred distinguished guests. Soon the double doors will open to a procession of diners more than ready to fill their plates and eat.

Chef steps back from the window and flicks the offending speck from an otherwise immaculate square of linen. He dabs at the sweat beaded on his forehead and the moisture above his lip. Like an actor before a big opening, he's memorized the entire play, from *escallopes de foie gras aux truffes* at one end of the buffet to a towering *meringues à la Chantilly* at the other. In between rests an extravagance of tricolored *terrines*, molten *gratins*, palate-bracing *tartares* and hand-tooled *patisseries*. His finest work, Chef dares to believe – each morsel a testament to the fertile marriage of artistry and food.

A dozen *garçons* in elegant black vests fall smartly in step as their leader strides from the kitchen, resplendent in a white coat and toque. He moves a sculpted radish a quarter-inch to the left, rotates a tray, inspects a flourish of intricately piped butters and icings. "*Bien,*" he says as the waiters strain to listen. "*Très bien!*"

Yet even as Chef inspects the laden tables, havoc is brewing in his hospitable counties of cuisine. Hosts of microscopic troublemakers — diaphanous rods, colonizing clusters, rare but tenacious rings and ribbons — are staking turf, unpacking toxins, sending lusty offspring out on juicy pathways to far reaches of tray, bowl and cutting board. Cooked in nature's kitchen, whole batches of uninvited thugs are getting ready to strike.

Chef examines an expanse of exquisite *hors-d'oeuvres* pureed and puffed to perfection and, *alors*, lavishly peppered with *Campylobacter*, a nasty unseen enteric villain recently arrived on the fecal-manual freeway via an infected *sous-chef* with inattentive hygiene. *Campylobacter* will cause fever, abdominal cramps and worse but not for two to five days, long after the oblivious dignitaries swallow their last *champignon farci*. Chef himself now transfers an outpost of *Campylobacter* from a silver tray to a white *serviette* by wiping up a spilled *soupçon* of *Béchamel*. In a subsequent flurry of polishing, he'll deposit those hardy voyagers inside a large bowl of shrimp.

Nearby, at the endive in the salad section, *Escherichia coli* has also recently arrived via the ever-efficient highway of unwashed hands. *Quel dommage! E. coli*, also known as *EC0157*, doubles its population every two hours and in the fecund territory of the buffet has prospered and multiplied. Already *EC0157* outnumbers the *crudités* by countless orders of magnitude and with every passing moment new generations mature. Soon endive-eating Honorables will encounter hemorrhagic colitis, an acute bloody diarrhea resembling dysentery that will make its presence known about the time the waiters circulate with the after-dinner *Courvoisier.*

While Chef and his followers continue their careful rounds, modest but growing portions of *Clostridium perfringens* and *Staphylococcus aureus* lie in wait among the *entrées* for passage on a fork or spoon to dark and devilish destinations. In the moist heat of the chafing dishes, these single-cell opportunists of untraceable origin are reproducing rapidly while natural selection sharpens their appetite for microscopic crime. *Personnages* who hoist *C. perfringens* or *S. aureus* to their lips will experience a pleasurable gustatory event followed by acute abdominal pain, nausea, and vomiting, regardless of rank.

On the dessert tray: *Listeria monocytogenes*. Although *L. monocytogenes* causes potentially fatal food poisoning and meningitis, only the smallest smidgen has survived its arduous journey from contaminated kitchen sponge to *mousse au chocolat*. In the romantic glow of the burning candelabra, this party pooper has begun its arithmetic dance – divide, multiply, divide – and may yet spread sufficiently to become the evening's *coup de grâce*.

As the evolutionary clock clicks forward, chimes ring throughout the crowded reception rooms. Chef strikes a pose near the rare roast beef while an elite corps of waiters stakes positions behind the buffet. *Les garçons*, the unwitting gardeners of this pathogenic smorgasbord, stand ready with sterling trowels and deceptive white towels to smooth gouges, fill gaps, mop errant droplets and generally tidy the 'hood for the bacterial gangs. Chef nods approvingly at a deft swipe of cloth by the innocent *jardinier* tending the ever more virulent *blanquette de veau*. Constant vigilance shall ensure that every *incroyable* dish on the buffet remains warm but not too warm, cold but not too cold, moist but not soggy, crisp where crisp is called for, plentiful and orderly through second and third helpings, multiple desserts, loquacious toasts — for hours on end — even as the last replete (and queasy) Under Secretary utters *adieu* and Chef himself sits down to dine.

Seconds tick ahead. Beads of candle wax slide into puddles on crystal *bobèches*. Chef fixes his attention on the closed double doors, his brow glistening with anticipation. Chimes sound again and the doors swing open. Chef dips his splendid toque in a heart-stopping bow and the distinguished dinner guests turn their heads and applaud.

COMPLEX CHOCOLATE CHOCOLATE COMPLEX

BY CHRIS CRITTENDEN

what is luscious
is what hurts is
what is measured
as it measures me

what is a seductress as slim
as an enticing camisole
on slippery hips

is what labels me
so ripe with calories
that i cannot be adequate

what is succulent
as a first kiss is what is
addictive as an endless one

what is precious is what
is cheap is what is so expensive
that i cannot run away from it
no matter where i buy spandex

VEGETABLE LOVE

BY BARBARA CROOKER

Feel a tomato, heft its weight in your palm,
think of buttocks, breasts, this plump pulp.
And carrots, fresh dirt clinging to the root,
gold mined from the earth's tight purse.
And asparagus, that push their heads through earth,
rise to meet the returning sun,
and zucchini, green torpedoes
lurking in the Sargasso depths
of their raspy stalks and scratchy leaves.
And peppers, thick walls of cool jade, a green hush.
Secret caves. Sanctuary.
And beets, the dark blood of the earth.
And all the lettuces: bibb, flame, oak leaf, butter-
crunch, black seeded Simpson, chicory, cos.
Elizabethan ruffs, crisp verbiage.
And spinach, the dark green
of northern forests, savoyed, ruffled,
hidden folds and clefts.

And basil, sweet basil, nuzzled
by fumbling bees drunk on the sun.
And cucumbers, crisp, cool white ice
in the heart of August, month of fire.
And peas in their delicate slippers,
little green boats, a string of beads,
repeating, repeating.
And sunflowers, nodding at night,
then rising to shout hallelujah! at noon.

All over the garden, the whisper of leaves
passing secrets and gossip, making assignations.
All of the vegetables bask in the sun,
languorous as lizards.

Quick, before the frost puts out
its green light, praise these vegetables,
earth's voluptuaries,
praise what comes from the dirt.

LUTEFISK WARS

BY LEE CUNNINGHAM

ix men in dazzling white shirts, sleeves rolled to near elbow, hunch over the battlefield. A chandelier reflects light from the new white oilcloth table cover, weighted down by sturdy restaurant-weight china and low profile glassware. The men wait quietly, their faces serious; they are ready for what they know will come.

Tension rides the warm air currents churned by children scampering to stay out of the way and women carrying loaded trays held high. Something else hangs heavy in the air. Steam from boiling water and a pungent mixture of smells roll out of the small kitchen where the dinner is almost ready for transport. Bowls and trays that haven't seen the light in a year are taken from the built-in corner cupboards in the dining room. Other bowls, reinforcements brought by relatives and tied in tea towels, and roasters wrapped in layers of newspaper to keep them warm, suffer denuding during these last moments before the scheduled attack.

The call – a Norwegian invitation to the table that sounds like *Veshigo* – goes out to everyone to take their positions. The men at the table move not a muscle. Small children herd each other into the guest bedroom and fight over little chairs grouped around little tables. Bigger children move into the privacy of the other bedroom where two card tables and grown-up chairs sit waiting.

The four sisters and the six wives of the warring brothers plan to sit around the kitchen table with all its leaves added. They mop their brows and ask each other if everything is out. The four brothers-in-law have a table in the living room flanking the dining room with a view through a wide archway.

Everyone is settled. Everything is ready. A hush falls. The oldest daughter gives the signal and the supply lines wind out of the kitchen. Three rush the big dining room table with two platters of *lutefisk*, two plates of folded *lefsa* and two bowls full of mashed potatoes topped with hollowed out craters full of melted butter, placing them strategically in synchronized action. The brothers study the terrain while they wait for the women's arms to retreat – the butter bearers, the water glass fillers, and the dish towel distributors. While yard-square dish towels are tied around the necks and draped carefully over the suit pants of each of the six brothers, they bite their lips, scratch their noses, rub their hands together – they're ready!

The attack begins when the oldest brother reaches for his first lefsa and scoops up a butter dish with the other hand. He moves his plate – which is only for supply storage – off to his right and toward the middle of the table and unfolds the velvety soft *lefsa*, carefully, you can be sure, covering a 15-inch circle on the table cloth. The butter slathering begins with a bricklayer's troweling action over the entire *lefsa* surface. Plops of mashed potatoes drop from giant spoons and skid around in the butter until they can be coaxed into a flat layer formation across the middle half of the circle.

Now, the celebrated *lutefisk* – this flesh of the codfish, lye-processed and water soaked many times, and boiled to a consistency somewhere between watermelon pickles and gelatin, then searched carefully for bones – is spread generously, reverently – over the mashed potatoes. The calloused and scarred hands of the oldest brother roll the first finished product – a long rolled burrito-style package about 15 inches long and fat, requiring both hands, strategically spread, to support the pliable delicacy. The tantalized oldest brother almost drools in anticipation as he lifts the delicate construction to his wide-open mouth. Five pairs of eyes watch to see if the *lefsa* succumbs or survives. *Lefsa* starts out as a mixture of riced potatoes, lard, and flour rolled out almost see-through thin and baked on the top of an old, seldom used now, wood-burning kitchen range fired hot with hardwood and maybe a speck or two of coal. A few brown spots and occasional air bubbles mark the finished product when it is ready to be lifted off the stovetop. None of this hard, hot work crosses the mind of any of these brothers at this long-anticipated moment.

The oldest brother gets the first delicious bite, of course. He always does. Encouraged by the fact his *lefsa* doesn't break, the elbows around the table fly, creating this annual tradition – serious and deadly as it is. The war is not over with the first bite of the first meal-in-a-*lefsa*. No – the contest ends when only one glutton is left at the table, having consumed more of these concoctions than any of the other five. They have strict rules about the butter slathering, potato troweling, *lutefisk* layering and *lefsa* rolling – and they count how much each consumes.

The oldest brother always wins. His strongest competition comes from Lloyd, the stutterer. Only one brother is not a true contender – the skinny alcoholic and smoker. The others all finish in order of their ages, the twins, the youngest, quitting first. The other brother loves to watch them and participates, but he does not eat to win. This ritual has gone on since they were all kids around this same table in a big farmhouse miles away. The issue is pride – like other men feel about playing chess with their sons. It's all over if the younger one wins.

What's at stake? A silly bet – something their mother does not know about. She would not approve. Each of the brothers has devoted his life to championing one breed of car. At this point in car evolution – the mid-1940s – they have huge arguments about the attributes of Ford, Dodge, Chevrolet, Buick, Pontiac, and Plymouth. The oldest brother can't afford to lose. His next car might have to be a Ford, cars he's been calling rattletraps for years. He'd rather be dead.

The other people in the house eat their dinners of butter-fried chicken, ham, meatballs, beef, sweet potatoes, mashed potatoes and chicken gravy, vegetables, fresh Parkerhouse rolls and kringles, baked beans, apple and mince pies, fruitcake, *sandbakkels,* rosettes, and ice cream – and maybe a little *lefsa* and *lutefisk,* especially the boys who are in training for the big table. Their moms clear their tables, steer the smallest kids into the bathroom to wash their hands, begin the dish washing and drying, and pray for the contest to be over soon.

The young boys and the brothers-in-law line the walls of the dining room, gasping over the outcome of this battle – the redness of faces, the bulging of eyes, and the undoing of zippers and buttons. An occasional fish bone works its way into the mouth of a warrior who maintains proper discipline, with no sympathy from the other five. Watching the young men looking at the older men, it is impossible for their mothers to tell if the IQ has improved or if this Norwegian Christmas folly will continue through another generation.

When the last white dish towel flag finally goes up, the winning and wounded warriors whale up into the lounger rockers and couches in the living room. Shirts are left unbuttoned, neckties lie abandoned on the field of battle, and zippers will probably never meet again on this day. An unplanned snoring contest ensues, unbeknown to the participants.

The youngest kids keep claim on the bathroom. Many of them don't have bathrooms in their homes yet, even though many have running water in their kitchens. Grandma's faucet with pressurized city water inspires creative minds that quickly discover the power of a small finger held over the faucet hole when the water's turned on. The water spurts and spray can be aimed at cousins. It can be held for a little while with no water coming out, but then – WOW! And it makes a great noise hitting the plastic shower curtain.

The other fascination is the clothes chute. To make the game really exciting, someone has to go down into the basement to be at the bottom of the chute. Anyone who has been conned into this job once never does it again. He will be spit upon, have water poured on him, and have hard objects dropped on his head – maybe even a small child who leans too far into the chute.

What can you expect from the children of six guys who eat themselves nearly to death every year to celebrate Christmas? And what can you expect from any group of people who enjoy the taste and smell of fish soaked in lye?* Not a lot more than standing on the toilet lid with a head in the clothes chute, spitting on cousins they see only once or twice a year and do not look forward to seeing again – except to get even!

---

* Editor's Note: Some say traditional *lutefisk* cod is first soaked in lye, then buried in the ground for six months, after which it is dug up, rinsed and boiled. Disparaging songs have been composed about the dish, with one published in the *Chicago Tribune* sung to the tune of the traditional holiday carol, "Oh, Christmas Tree"; the first line of The *Lutefisk* Song goes, "Oh *lutefisk*, oh *lutefisk* – your smell is so disgusting..." The debate continues.

THESE OLD PANS

BY JOANNE DALBO

ow do you go from rolling dough to rolling tar? Let's just say that Dad could think outside of the box. Whether my dad worked as a baker or a roofing contractor, he was always a baker. As a little child, I remember hearing the creak of the door as he left the house in the small hours of the morning to go to his job at Pride Bakery. I pictured him, with his strong, thick hands, kneading the dough that he would turn into large hearty loaves of bread or small delicate pastries. I imagined him looking out the window into the darkness of the early morning where street lights shone on parked cars in front of red brick houses with black windows, the inhabitants still sleeping while this big, gentle man carefully prepared the sweets they would savor with their coffee.

When rolling dough no longer provided the salary to feed and clothe his growing family, my dad climbed the financial ladder to the lucrative occupation of roofing contractor. This change in career did not stop the baking. The small oven in our kitchen began to boast of the most elegant treats. Often, every corner of our kitchen caught and held the warm smell of baking. In October, our kitchen's breath smelled of sweet apples; in the deep winter, the stirring scent of dough baking rose from long, golden brown loaves of Italian bread – aromatherapy before it became a marketable product. As the pies cooked, he lined up more pie tins – silver, with little holes in the bottom. He peeled the furry skin of the peaches with a small sharp knife, slicing the fruit into mile-high piles. He trimmed the extra dough from the sides of the pie pans and elegantly fluted the edges with his big hands. I watched with the wonder of a child as a seemingly endless number of pies went into and slid out of our oven.

"Dad, how can you cut up so many peaches, make so many pies?"

"You don't think about the whole job. You just think about the one thing you have to do right now."

When Dad made pizza, he lined up the long, heavy, flat pizza pans. Though well scrubbed, they carried the black scars of many years of baking. I can still see my father's muscles move in his forearms as he kneaded and punched the dough down into the deep stainless steel bowls. He covered them with clean kitchen towels while the dough slowly rose under his loving gaze. The smell of bubbling tomato sauce invited droves of aunts, uncles, cousins and friends to our table to take that first bite into the crispy, then soft, crust with just a touch of olive oil. The kitchen filled with the sound of talk, the kind that people enjoyed before television drew them away. Our many gatherings became informal dinner theatres, as I come from a generation of storytellers. We sat around the table either telling or listening to tales, some true, some spiced with just the right amount of seasoning. My father baked stories into his pastries and pies. He knew just the right ingredients to whet and satisfy the appetites of his guests.

◇ ◇ ◇

Now, my mother doesn't know what to do with all these old pans since dad passed away just this past January. She wants to keep a few, but 30? As she wonders out loud, I look at the collage of pictures on the wall and my gaze locks on to a photo of my father, 14 years old, decorating a wedding cake. In my house, already cramped and filled with "stuff," I know I have to find room for these old pans. I begin to panic about when I'm going to find the time to organize all that "stuff" in my house. Then I remember Dad's peach pies and decide I'm just going "to think about the one thing I have to do right now."

GROWING UP FAT

BY E.-K. DAUFIN

Growing up fat,
too many ig'nant boyz
& my family,
didn't know I was fine,
The dogs preferred chasing bones to an extra helping of
femme fatale divine.

It used to hurt.
I wasted precious time,
Learning how to
fake laughing it off,
Heal, hurt, cry and whine,
But now the bad boyz
who too stupid to
'preciate
My big, beautiful design,
can break their teeth on bones,
Eat the sh-t they can't
tell from shinola,
And *don't* get the pleasure
of kissing my big, soft,
Lickable, lovable
fragrant,
flagrantly fat,
bodacious behind!

Why have a little
when you can have a lot?
Get to steppin', you minus 10-IQ,
anorexic lovin' (P-U!),
sheep-minded lot,
Thin may be in,
But fat is what's hot.

You got to have you some fat
if you fittin' to fry.
Are you a breast man?
Or do you prefer a plump thigh?

MISS TISH AND THE OKREE LADIES

BY TISH DAVIDSON

umid air wrapped me in its clammy embrace, leaving a glaze of sweat on my forehead even though it was only seven on this August morning in 1978. The air stank of rotting vegetation. Randolph Trappey, a graying, jowly man, reached out his hand to escort me across the rush of water from an overflowing potato peeler. The rattle of empty cans and the grumble of heavy equipment made conversation impossible.

The B. F. Trappey's Sons cannery in Lafayette, Louisiana, had been founded in 1893 by Randolph's grandfather. Randolph, called Mr. Randolph by everyone from the janitor to the plant foreman, still lived in a house about a hundred yards from the factory. Although half a dozen family members were active in the company, he was the driving force behind the family business.

I had arrived in Lafayette three months before, a new bride with a husband in graduate school. I needed a job, any job. After several interviews, Mr. Randolph, under extreme pressure from his plant foreman to fill the job, reluctantly made me an offer to head the quality control department. He told me straight out that he'd rather hire a man, but that he was desperate for a college graduate to take the job.

Moving along the corridor to an unmarked door, Mr. Randolph held it open for me. A blast of gloriously cool air hit us as we entered the quality control lab that would be my domain for the next two years.

"Ladies," said Mr. Randolph, "This here is Mrs. Davidson, your new boss."

Their work interrupted, they stood before me — the elite of the women cannery workers, the quality control morning shift — Lizzie Trahan, Marie Richard, Vivian Bourque, Mary Broussard, and Marlene Hebert. Soon I would meet the rest of the lab ladies, as they called themselves — 14 women in all. Most were old enough to be my mother, a few old enough to be my grandmother. Starting that day, they were all working under the supervision of a 25-year-old stranger with a newly minted Ivy League degree and zero experience in management.

Once Mr. Randolph left the lab, it became apparent that I was an alien invader. Not only had I dropped in from Planet Nawth, I spoke a foreign language – English. In the years before Paul Prudhômme put Cajun spices in cupboards across America, Cajun culture existed in an inbred, tightly circumscribed triangle in southwest Louisiana. Well into the 1960s it remained protected from outsiders by bayous swarming with alligators, nutria, mosquitoes, and a distinct lack of anything the outside world could covet. Every woman over 35 in the Trappey lab grew up speaking Cajun French at home, school, and church, and still conducted her daily affairs with Cajun French as her first, and often her only, fluent language.

◇ ◇ ◇

The first few weeks on the job staggered by in a blur of noise and headaches. Although I had youth and education on my side, it was clear from the start that I couldn't tell a Number 10 can from a 303. Two shifts were canning okra, universally called okree, and sweet potatoes, universally called yams. Fortunately, the lab ladies, although they were almost all high school dropouts, knew the routine. They gently ignored me and did what needed to be done, no matter how often I got in their way.

Occasionally someone would approach me, diffidently calling me Miss Tish, and tell me things that I was supposed to know. This was the Trappey version of on-the-job training. But mostly the lab ladies kept busy sampling, measuring, counting, timing, weighing, and chatting endlessly in a guttural French that sounded so unlike my university-learned version that I was not sure it was the same language. The lab ladies were never impolite, insubordinate, angry, or difficult, but try as I might, I couldn't get more than a polite nod or a deferential, "Yes, Miss Tish," out of any of them before they continued their endless rounds of work and conversation.

◇ ◇ ◇

One day, after about three weeks on the job, heavy, lumbering Lizzie Trahan opened the first crack in the communication wall. Looking up from weighing a No. 10 can of yams, and apropos to nothing, she spoke to me, in English. "Do you make your rice sticky or plain?"

Sticky or plain? I hardly ever made any kind of rice, coming from a Pennsylvania Dutch family of devoted potato eaters. Sticky or plain? Was this some kind of initiation? Fortunately Lizzie gave me a clue. "When my husband was in the service, we lived in Hawaii next to a Japanese family. They made their rice sticky. Do you make yours sticky or plain?"

"Plain," I answered gratefully.

"Do you fry your okree or smother it?"

"Actually, I've never had okra, I mean okree."

All movement in the lab stopped.

"Never had okree. Child!" Lizzie looked as appalled as if I had just told her that I stewed baby brains and ate them for lunch.

By the time the shift whistle blew at 4 PM, half the factory, the female half, knew that Tish Davidson, Quality Control Director, had never eaten okree.

The next morning during a break, Lizzie waddled over to me with a plastic container. "Here," she puffed. "Made you some smothered okree last night. Taste it."

"Great." I tasted the mixture of okra, tomatoes, and onions. "Yum." It really was good. "How did you make this, Lizzie?"

Mary Broussard bustled in. "Miss Tish," she said, "we had smothered okree last night. I brought you some."

"Yum, great."

A little while later rigid, angular Marie Richard appeared and shyly held out a container and a fork. "Everyone should know how to make smothered okree," she said.

Before the day was over, half a dozen versions of smothered okree had passed my lips, and I had made a solemn vow to each of the cooks that I would go home and make smothered okree for my Jewish, New York City husband. "You got to learn cookin', if you don't want dat boy leavin' you," said Blanche Thibodeaux, the line supervisor.

A few days later Lizzie appeared with another container. "Gumbo," she said. "Sausage and chicken."

"Better with duck," said Judy Duplechain, the water quality girl who happened to be passing through the lab.

"Crawfish," said tiny Lynne Leger.

"Squirrel gumbo got more flavor," insisted Marie Richard.

The next day samples appeared, fortunately none with squirrel.

During the following weeks I was given careful instructions on how to make a dark roux without burning it, how to pick the fat out of the heads of crawfish for *étouffée*, how to butcher a turtle, how to skin a frog. The women in my lab were genuinely concerned that I had been allowed to enter the state of holy wedlock without learning these things. The fact that I could make the dishes of my grandmothers — *snitz* and *knepp*, apple fritters, shoo fly pie, and chow chow - didn't count as being able to cook. They fretted that my husband, "dat boy" they always called him, would leave me for a girl who knew her jambalaya.

◇ ◇ ◇

One day Mary, the most articulate of the group, asked me what food from "up Nawth" I got hungry for. "Pig stomach," I said picking the most outlandish Pennsylvania Dutch dish I could think of.

As I described the dish to Mary — a pig stomach, cleaned and stuffed with potatoes, sausage, and onions, then roasted to a crispy brown — she started to smile. *"Chaudette,"* she said. "Dat's what we Cajuns call it. Only we put rice in, 'steada Irish potatoes. You fix *chaudette* for dat boy of yours, you gonna be okay. Maybe you Yankees don't be so dumb after all."

LIFT A GLASS OF DAGO RED
BY ALBERT DEGENOVA

Louie Prima on the stereo
gets my foot tappin'
gets my pulse poundin'
    like espresso sweetened with anisette,
makes me remember dago red
(the pride of Italian immigrant grandpas
who cut their homemade wine with orange juice
for us 9-year-olds)
remember all those Sunday dinners
the shot of vermouth to start
the *provolone* and *pepperoni,*
mostaccioli with thick red sauce
and the gravy meat
meatballs, *brociols,* chunks of pork,
then a roast beef
fresh green beans, corn
baked potatoes
tomatoes from the garden with herbs and olive oil
where we dipped hard crust bread hot out of the oven
remember dessert cakes
and cookies and then
the dark, dark coffee
and shots of sweet liqueur,
kick back the rugs
spin the black vinyl
and dance and laugh
and dance and laugh
and laugh
and eat
"*mangia, mangia*"
Sunday at Grandma's
the Old Country on the tips of our tongues.
Oh, for another glass
of that dago red!

PYGGY PYGGY
(A PORCINE VERSION of WILLIAM BLAKE'S "TYGER TYGER")
BY STAR DONOVAN

Pyggy, pyggy, glowing bright
On the spitfire grill tonight
With puckered snout and curly tail,
Delicious with a pint of ale.

Bacon, ham and pork chops, too
There's enough for all of you
Sausage, stew, four knuckles and
The best darn trotters in the land.

Crispy fat doth pop and fry
Gather round to sniff and sigh,
For crackling we shall have galore.
Just one bite, you'll ask for more.

Cholesterol? We do not care!
Of heart attacks we are aware,
But pork just tastes so good to eat
We can't resist such tasty meat!

A splash of gravy on the plate
'taters, veg, it's not too late,
So bring your bread and bring your bun
'cause this ol' pyggy's just on done.

Pyggy, wyggy, roasting right
On the spitfire grill tonight
Add some sprouts and curly kale,
Delicious with a pint of ale.

THE CHICAGO HOT DOG POEM:
ODE TO FLUKY'S, POOCHIES, AND WOLFY'S

BY CHERIE CASWELL DOST

the one time
I ordered a hot dog
in the state of California
the clerk asked me
"Skin or no skin?"

I answered
with the sound
of the door
finding the door frame
again

TEA AT MY GRANDMOTHER'S

ROBERT KLEIN ENGLER

old stipples the rim of the china cup I bring to my lips. The old radio, turned to Chopin, plays softly from its cove of shadows near the sofa. Some pears glow with a ripe blush in their blue bowl set over a doily. The cat pads across the floor to pause and look up at me, then passes on to its cushion by the bay window. Grandmother offers me a scone with a gesture that stammers at the end of its arc like the static from the antique Zenith. How her eyes are like my mother's eyes; something with the blue of a jewel, or the sky, or the lake painted topaz over white. The tea tastes of earth and of parchment written with lamb's blood. I listen to her slow words. She adds another pearl to the string that unwinds from one closed room to another. Albums of mummy leather pass from hand to hand. "From a long way off you remember the shape of love," she says, "but not its song." I look out to the street where the new world parades with the burden of a rose. Have you seen it, rain falling into sunlight? So is the sorrow inside joy.

POETRY BUFFET

BY JO LEE DIBERT-FITKO

I have covered my table with the
delicacy of fine woven linen,
polished silver's shining enunciations.
You arrive with butter-dripping words,
warm French bread whose crusty shell collapses
to soft center's eagerness.

Tender crumbs playfully
licked reveal porcelain smooth speech,
tease hunger's mounting appetite.
Tangy juices released from
your lingual fruits are sweet desserts,
secretive trespassers.

I scoop you up in emotion's frosting,
spread you delectably thin
or gushing whipped thickness.
Confection samplers of
savory verse promise always
a ripened abundance.

Just buffet me.
Quench the thirsty cup.
Drip seductively that
rich mellowing cream of language.
Entice me.
I'll be the spoon arousing slowly,
waltzing gently through
your dark strong
coffee
            waiting.

PASTA

BY BARRY FRAUMAN

Sensual slide over tongue and lips,
a shame we have to chew our noodles.
For greater taste, oil, spices and sauce,
but oh that voluptuous pasta glide!

Italian is my favorite food,
but some Chinese noodles are sexy-smooth;
and then my background, Russian Jewish:

varéniki, pale ravioli
filled with cherries or blueberries,
best dessert my grandmother made.
Another treat, *kugel* (G hard),
was broad baked noodles
with cottage cheese, egg, salt and pepper.
Mother and Grandmother made it that way.
My father's stepmother wrecked the dish
with pineapple, raisins, maraschinos.
I wasn't a kid to O.D. on sugar,
not with a dish alongside meat.
Unfortunately, this too-sweet *kugel*
is featured in every delicatessen.
The salt-and-pepper? Mother's recipe?
Dare I guess?

MOVE OVER, DARWIN

BY DIANNE L. FRERICHS

'm not exactly the food police. The food police are those that harass you about five fruits and vegetables a day or how much saturated fat or sodium you are consuming. They sneak around and pop up when you least expect them. That is not me.

I am also not exactly religious about food, either. You know those people. And God created broccoli, cauliflower, and Brussels sprouts and said, "Enjoy." And Satan brought forth hot fudge and chocolate chip cookies and said, " Want to really enjoy, little girl?" Then God created tofu, bean sprouts, and rice cakes and said, "Be full of nourishment and enjoy." Satan responded with, "Psst, over here. You two – red meat, and double baked potatoes with sour cream and decadent chocolate cheesecake. Live it up!" I'm not them, either.

What I am, I guess, is a food historian or, more accurately, a gastronomic anthropologist. I want to know the origins and I have begun to work out a theory.

Back at the beginning of time, when hominids first appeared, they relied on the other animals for food. They watched. Crouching in their caves, they peered out at the wilds to see what was a viable food source. They watched to see what seeds, nuts, berries and fruits the bird-like creatures would eat. And they followed suit. Rather like the birds and the bush next to my house.

Each spring it is covered with dark purple berries and the birds adore them. They come from miles around to gorge themselves on those berries. They then proceed to poop blue-purple bird crap all over my neighbor's house, car, and driveway. After relieving themselves, the birds come back for more and the cycle continues. Fruit – crap – more fruit, until all the berries are gone. I can imagine early man facing that. It may be one of the primary reasons they were nomadic, changing caves frequently. What a joy without Charmin!

So that's how food choices must have begun, by watching other animals. The carnivores showed early man what meat to eat and how to kill it. But I'm quite sure that the earliest humanoids fought for the leftovers of the other meat-eaters. Carrion is not on my list, but back then maybe it was palatable.

But what about food that is fine for animals but dangerous for people? There are poisonous plants and animals like that. In addition to certain leaves and berries, there are venomous critters that can endanger or even kill a human being while not doing damage to other forms of animal life. Was that part of the survival of the fittest? The part nobody mentions? Eat poisonous food and you exit the gene pool. But food doesn't end with observational dining.

I believe the next great step in the evolution of food was fire. Lightning struck the forest and fire rushed through, burning all in its wake. Ta-dah! – Roasted meat and roasted vegetables. Mankind ate well that day and learned. And that was the birth of man's love for Weber grills.

But the gnawing question has always been who was the Edison of food? Who put what together and who ate it first? How did certain fundamental foods come into existence? Who first ground cereals into flour and how did they decide to do that? Did a rock fall on a cereal stalk and an early Edison saw the pulverization? He then continued pounding to see what would happen. Did he notice the bubbling fermentation in some puddle of smashed grain and say, "Let's see what happens when we push it together with our hands and roll it around then add heat?" Was that the birth of bread? And could a variation on this theme have been the reaction of smashed fruit to the bubbling? The final result being giggle juice.

And who first consumed the new concoctions? I have discovered the answer. There is a sub-species of human that has been developed. They are either dumb as a rock or brave beyond belief. I have named these omnivorous humanoids Mikey Pithicus. For generations, they have been food testers. From pre-history food creation through the Dark Ages of royal food tasters, Mikey Pithicus has been there. They have spread throughout the world to all lands and cultures. Even now their descendants are employed by a breakfast food company, where we once again hear the cry, "Let Mikey try it. He'll eat anything!"

So from time immemorial, food has developed by accident or experiment and there have been those who tried it. We owe our lives and our dining pleasures to those food Edisons and the Mikeys of history.

BREAD

BY VINCENT F. A. GOLPHIN

The smell shifts through the rooms
    Of the house where I was born
        Like my mother who never stayed in the kitchen.

One room could not hold the Virginia rolls,
    A handed-down recipe
        That smelled of long-past times and places.

Baked barely brown,
    Darkest on the mounded crest,
    A rich yellow cast around the tan edges.
The soft substance melted in buttery bites
    Pressed between my tongue
        And the roof of my mouth
    Rolled comfort and security
        Into every aroma-charged chamber.
Like the baker
    Who breezed from room to room,
        Touching and fixing,
    While the doughy memories stretched
    Until they covered every hall.

They became one with everything that was good
    About my childhood.
Rolls the size of my grown, right hand,
    Pulled, Pounded, Plucked and Shaped,
        By yellow-brown fingers that seemed too small
            To make a difference, in many ways,
            Except, like the smell of those rolls
            They wrought my joy when I was a boy.

MR. BRADLEY'S BAR-B-Q

BY VINCENT F.A. GOLPHIN

The sharp, sour vinegar smell,
laced with enough lemon to notice,
washed across the landscape of my green grass playground.

A sign of spring
    more reliable than the birds,
    or the lengthening warmth of the sun,
    it trailed in gray-blue smoke.

Mr. Bradley turned pork ribs (never beef or chicken)
    into a glazed, burnt-red death celebration,
    but never invited a guest.

The roast made passersby and neighbors lust
    for meat that smelled good enough
    to make a sow's death a privilege.

HUNGRY ANNA

BY SUSAN HANNUS

hen I opened the newspaper, I saw a picture of an old, frail, gray-haired woman with metal-rimmed glasses. Having recently lost my beloved grandfather, this caught my eye. The article was about a 92-year-old woman named Anna. It told about her experiences with a senior meal-delivery plan. She stated that it wasn't enough food, and that it wasn't very edible. In fact, she said she was often hungry.

I couldn't believe what I was reading. I put down the newspaper, and got out my phone book. The only listing for her last name, on that street, was for a man named John. I took a chance that it was her late husband's name and called the number. The old woman's voice on the other end confirmed that it was indeed Anna. I spent the next half-hour talking to her, and she invited me to her home the following day.

As I turned onto her street, I became very nervous. What would I say to her? What could I do for this poor woman? After parking my car, I walked up her cracked cement stairs and rang the bell. It took about five minutes before the heavy wooden door creaked open. She looked like her picture, a small, bent-over woman with wire rimmed glasses, and her hair a gray-yellow, twisted in a bun, held back by black bobbie pins. When I stepped into her living room, the smells of an old person's house assaulted me: perspiration, Ben Gay, stale air and mothballs. We sat for a while talking. I told her about my family and myself. She told me she was glad "someone" cared. A teakettle in the next room was whistling. I asked her if I could make the tea. She told me the tea bags were in the cookie jar on the counter. As I entered the kitchen, I saw pile after pile of food containers, milk cartons, and rotting fruit. There must have been five unwrapped sandwiches. It was difficult for me to walk back into the living room with the tea. I tried to compose myself before asking her about all that food.

Her explanation to me was that "it was all wrong." They brought her a hot meal at noon and a sandwich for dinner. She did not *like* eating a hot meal at noon. So she left the food on the counter and then it *wasn't any good* by dinnertime. And the sandwich was usually turkey, and she *hated* turkey. The only time she could *bear* to eat a sandwich was when it was ham. The fruit they brought her was *always overripe*, and she *never* ate overripe fruit. I could hardly listen to her complaining. When I asked her if she ever told them about her concerns, she pruned up her face and said, "The delivery man is a Negro, and I don't speak to Negroes."

At home that afternoon, I thought about my grandfather. He was a simple man with few demands. How lucky I was to have had him. He never would have complained about turkey instead of ham, and I never heard my grandfather speak ill of people who were different. But I was determined to make a dent in this woman's way of thinking, so the next week I called on her again.

When I arrived at her house, there was an elderly woman leaving. I stopped to introduce myself to her. The woman told me not to think I could get anything from Anna. I politely told her my name and why I was there, but she sniffed the air and turned from me and walked away. I talked to Anna about her. She told me her neighbor, Sophie, shopped for her every week and did her laundry, too. With some hesitation I asked her about her remarks in the newspaper about being alone. Certainly, Sophie was company for her. When she spoke of Sophie, she made a face as if she had been forced to eat turkey. She told me that Sophie was *only after* her antique rocking chair, and that the *only* reason *that* woman shopped for her was because she hoped to get that chair. She *never* promised Sophie that chair, but she let her think it was a possibility; otherwise Sophie might charge her for doing her shopping.

I walked into her kitchen and not only saw the abundance of food containers, but some big cardboard boxes. I asked her about them, and she stiffened when she told me they had come in the mail. Inside the opened boxes were canned soups, beans, jellies, peanut butter, oatmeal and cookies. It seemed that many people were moved by her story of hunger. *If they only knew,* I said to myself. I told her it was wonderful that people had cared so much. She snapped at me that she was *not* a charity case, and besides she *didn't like* what they had sent her. I reminded her that she told the newspaper how hungry she was and how little money she had. At that, she took her cane and knocked a pile of letters off her desk. With haughtiness in her voice, she told me that *those people* thought she was looking for a handout, too. As I looked at each letter, I was deeply touched by the sentiments in them, and surprised by the generous checks and cash inside.

But the most touching letter of all was from two men from Skokie, Illinois. They had read about her plight in the paper. In their letter they said she was the same age as their mother – if their mother had survived the Holocaust. They had sent her a check for two hundred dollars, in honor and memory of their mother. When she saw me reading that letter, she raised her voice at me and said, "They think I am Jewish! I'm Polish! I don't want *their* money!" Her cruel words unnerved me. How could bigotry and racism be wrapped up into such a harmless looking package?

I stood up and put on my coat. As I walked toward the door, I turned around to look at her. Had those people wasted their kindness on her? Is kindness ever wasted? "Anna," I said, "you were right. You are starving."

I shut the door behind me and went home to feed my family.

SOUL FOOD

BY JULIA MORIS-HARTLEY

artinis: A few nights ago, I went to a banquet, an annual party thrown by my good friend Frankie, a swanky, fast-talker. I'd spent an entire month's savings to buy the pale blue silk gown that I wore, and another month's to buy Frankie his present, a portrait of him done by my up-and-coming artist boyfriend, Tony. I slicked my short hair back, tight against my head, so that it wouldn't whip in my eyes as I carried the huge brown parcel around the piazza while I searched for Tony, who'd come early to help Frankie get ready. There were 30 round tables, each set for four, arranged in a circle around the dance floor in the piazza's main hall; candles glittered, making flames of the crystal wineglasses. Star jasmine wafted through open windows, and a string quartet played out in the courtyard: the occasional tips of their bows incised the air beyond the French doors. I found Tony sitting at the bar with Dean. He smiled. "Doll! Don't you look beautiful tonight!"

I gave him a big kiss for noticing. "Gee, thanks, Ton. You don't look so bad yourself..." Boy, did he ever look good. He wore a black tux, black jacquard vest underneath, and a burgundy bow tie; his baby blues sparkled with mischief. He lifted the parcel from my arms, setting it on the floor against the bar. Then, he put his arm around my waist and we went looking for our table. His hand felt warm and electric on my back. Frankie, he said, winking, could find the present later.

Dean and his girl, Maxine, shared the table with us. She had a bubbly laugh and giggled increasingly as she drank more wine. Tony and I ordered martinis. Dean told one-liners until we were giddy and our sides hurt. Dinner was delicious, seven courses: poached northern salmon, orange ginger duck, red and black Beluga, slicelets of *foie gras*, baby butter leaf salad, chocolate *mousse*, bread so soft it melted on your tongue, and of course goblets and goblets of wine. Frankie gave a speech before and after we ate, getting out of his seat every now and again to sing one of his songs and coo at all the girls. After dinner, Tony and I sidled up to the bar and drank two more martinis. Natalie and Robert stumbled by, arms linked and eyes transfixed on one another. Tony started humming "I'm in the Mood for Love," and swept me onto the dance floor. I was in heaven. We danced a couple of circles around the dance floor, receiving applause from all sides. Sammy Jr. puffed on his cigar and winked at me. "Oh, Ton – what a girl!"

Tony smiled and pulled me tighter. He whispered, "You're great, baby doll." I laughed and looked up in time to see Dean, who caressed my elbow and flourished me away from my man, the up-and-coming Mr. Bennett.

✪

Later, I found Tony at his place at Mar-a-Lago. Somehow, he looked older, more mischievous. Even his brunette hair seemed to be going white. I hadn't gone to sleep and I'd had several martinis. He picked up what looked like a book from the table by the terrace. It was a canvas. Shocked, I gasped, as he rotated the canvas for me to see; this was Tony's secret side, which he'd refused to reveal to me. It was a painting that he'd done of us dancing at the banquet. The only two figures I could clearly make out were our own; everyone else was part of a darkened blur, an Impressionist jumble of periphery. A light illuminated us that had not been there while we danced, save for the light in his eyes.

"Tony..." I began, but could not find the words. I stared at the painting. "It's *beautiful*."

"Thanks, doll. Don't you ever forget that Tony loves you." He kissed my forehead and I cried. I think that might have been the happiest night of my life, except I dreamt it all after drinking two martinis and falling asleep to "Isn't It Romantic?" When I awoke the smell of wax lingered in the air and I tasted vodka on my lips. A blue bird flew past my window, its wings unfurling like a long blue dress and the sun bright as the twinkle in Tony Bennett's eyes.

✪ ✪ ✪

Olives: He passed before I got a good look at him. I only saw the uneven rise of his stride, the overshot ups and fluid, lolling downs. He wore a black fedora with a white ribbon. Black tee shirt, tucked in, and dyed shorts, whitewashed and thick-seamed, that reached his knees, where he'd rolled up the hem. Thin, bare legs tapered to thin, sock-clad ankles and yellowing canvas shoes that seemed too small tapped out an arrhythmic beat against the long, brown tiled hallway. I listened as he walked out of sight: Bum—ba-bum—ba—bum.

I can only imagine the stranger's face: large, brown eyes, looking sad beneath bifocal lenses; Roman nose, a long, aquiline lambda, two flared and symmetrical nostrils; thin, purplish lips pursed as if to catch the little beads of sweat forming on his upper lip and moistening his hairline. I imagine a half-hearted mustachio, sallow cheeks, and olive skin.

He must have been a dark baby. He must have come from some Aegean country, some salt-crusted, reefed beach along the Mediterranean, where figs grow and olive trees blossom yellow in the spring. People from that region recognize the poetic sensuality of the olive, how it pleases all the senses: not only is it round and firm to the touch, its texture is decadent on one's tongue, and its aroma and flavor are unmistakable. The olive begins life sour and puckered; brine cultivates the olive, making the fruit look lovely and inviting in any dish, but especially when placed along one's lips: soft pink flesh draws out the potency and allure of the olive's shape. This stranger must have come from a scorching Mediterranean place and felt the heavy, intertwined roots of the olive tree connected somehow to his soul.

I have seen the Mediterranean only in pictures: huge red nets spread over weather-beaten fishing boats; colonies of cats waiting at the docks for fishermen who return with buckets of small fish; long blue stairways ascending the hills, dividing rows of white houses.

My brother once visited Greece for some months. He fell in love with the starkness of the land, the white of the beaches, the cool, pale water. He drank a lot of ouzo. While in Greece, he sent me pictures of Santorini and Mikonos: huge expanses of white and sudden portals of unabashed color − cobalt, crimson, marigold, violet. His skin shone, dark and tan, and the sun bleached the tips of his hair white-gold. In photos, my brother stands proud, some new god in front of the white walls, smiling with abandon at the sound of distant drums: Bum—ba-bum—ba—bum.

◇ ◇ ◇

Garlic: Folk medicine was not wholly incorrect when it first engendered the notion that garlic wards off vampires. It wards off most other frightening things. Certainly, garlic thwarts cancers and weak immune systems; it also promotes healthier blood pressure and builds stronger, more discerning palates. Garlic, collected in its frail, translucent sac, is like a bundle of gems, collected for the celebration of long life.

A lesser-known bit of folklore decrees that two people predisposed to garlic should never fall in love. Like most Mediterranean gems, garlic is a hot weather creation, dependent on heat to release its juices and reach the apex of its flavor. Two hot weathered people eating roasted garlic engage in a highly combustible activity, due at any time to explode.

I've roasted countless pots of those aromatic clusters in the oven – how the oil popped and crackled as it infused the hot cloves! While the garlic roasted, I envisioned long rows of grapevines sloping the Italian Alps as some young man named Sandro or Niccolo walked desolately amongst them, whistling Italian folk songs and day-dreaming of the poetry in a woman's naked form. Oh, Niccolo, I wondered, why are you so elusive?

When finally Niccolo entered my life, he may have changed his name, but I recognized his song and slipped gratefully on an oily garlic skin into his poetic and crazy arms.

I knew he had mental problems before I started dating him. I'd sat in his office – an expansive music library at the radio station where I worked – numerous times, where he confided to me his certainty that he heard what the neighbors were saying about him, even their whispers; his conviction that his ex-girlfriend drove by his house every day to show off her (many) new boyfriends; his failure to successfully commit suicide. He talked and I listened and one day I found myself sitting on his lap, my hands hopelessly tangled in his long, dark hair, kissing his lips like my own life depended on it. I chanted his name like a mantra... John.

He lived in a Brooklyn neighborhood north of Kings Plaza, in a two-bedroom apartment that he shared with a roommate who was almost never there. A typical trip to his house involved 45 minutes on the subway and another half-hour on a lethargic bus, whose slow, lurching movements would often lull me into a drowse. John met me at the bus stop and we walked the 10 or so blocks to his brownstone, then up two flights of stairs. He cracked jokes the whole way.

But the entire neighborhood was sluggish; people dragged themselves about as if half-asleep, as if their limbs weighed more than they could bear. We were in one of New York's five boroughs, and the streets were so silent and barren that we felt alone. The mood followed us into his apartment. We didn't do much — watched television, cooked elaborate Italian dishes, drank too much red wine and smoked a lot — and he sat near me at all times, chuckling softly, telling me he loved me, asking me not to go. The sparse living room absorbed his words, leaving thick silence around us.

At night, in his bed, the orange street lights lit the ceiling and cast shadows of our clothes. If it rained, we heard an occasional car slide by or maybe a stray honk; if it was early in the evening, we sometimes heard conversations outside. John lay next to me, smelling of smoke, sweat, and garlic, the sound of his breathing an extension of the rain.

Once I dared ask if he could still hear what his neighbors said. "Yes," he said, swallowing. I could tell that he shut his eyes.

"What are they saying?" I asked.

"They're saying what a loser I am, how I don't deserve you, how you're gonna leave me."

I kissed him then and, foolish thing that I was, asked if he could still hear them. After a lengthy pause, he said "yes" again, more painfully.

We stayed together for the duration of a year, and I rarely realized that what was going on in my head was not the same as what was going on in his. Sometimes, though, I did realize and it caught me by surprise — I could forget his demons and torments and envision John as an ideal companion. But he could not forsake his demons and in the end the voices correctly predicted our inevitable separation. I got a job in another state and moved away; he chose not to come with me, preferring the sleepy neighborhood where his family still lived. He was in his late twenties and had a good job.

Some 8,000 years ago, the Mediterranean Sea flooded the Caspian Sea, which later became the Crimea and still later the Black Sea. When the flood subsided, the two seas separated, receding to their original corners of the world. I suppose that all things happen for such reasons, including the separation from John: garlic lovers as we were, doomed to temperamental flights of fancy and connected by a secret deluge several thousand years old. Garlic has since become less integral to my cooking, perhaps because I realize its potent sting. Each time I smell garlic now, my eyes water and I want to scream out his name: Hey John, come to dinner! Hey John, what went wrong? And then I think of his kisses and wonder quietly, John... John... Can you still hear them?

◇ ◇ ◇

Juniper: He went to Polynesia with the girl who should have been me.

He bought me a dress on our first date. And peeled naked out of a wetsuit on our second. He wanted me to meet his cool hippie friend who lived on the mountain by Bear Lake; its cerulean expanse glittered as we drove alongside. He ogled me at a friend's wedding while I smoked cigarettes outside with professors, my father's peers, and I begged them not to tell. When he smiled, I heard the ringing of far-off wind chimes.

He broke my heart in triplicate, peeling back each layer with thin, deft strokes: once saying I was too young, twice with the phone numbers I found scrawled on bar matchbooks next to his bed, and finally, leaving just when I felt closest to him.

Still, he appeared on my birthday, offering me a mashed potato smiley face on a stolen kitchen plate. I trembled all afternoon.

When I worked in a local market, we kept herbs and spices in gleaming Kerr jars. There, tucked between Indian Spice and Kudzu, we kept a small jar of dried juniper berries, which we sold for the hefty sum of roughly $4.00 per ounce. The shriveled berries sold very slowly. Occasionally, I liked to walk by the juniper jar, unscrew its lid, and inhale the spicy perfume. After him, I left the jar alone. Sometimes I envision him back in Logan Canyon, poised on all fours atop a patched, black inner tube, his hair drizzling wet against his forehead. He bobs in the current, laughing. I hear that laugh even today and turn around suddenly, only to see the river and China Rock through juniper brambles: dark, pungent berries obscure him as he drifts downstream, yelling, "Come on!"

BED OF LETTUCE

BY JULEY HARVEY

passing lettuce-pickers
in the fields,
midwife deliverers
of the newborn,
red-crying strawberries,
all the growing lusty lovelies
that come to grace our tables,
no matter the season or weather,
earth-babies,
brought forth from hunger-hands,
california's corn-husked,
grape-wrathed cornucopia
tumbles out of the jumbled, dusty days
of *juans* and *rosalitas*,
kerchiefed, hatted, sun-browned
the colors of earth,
and paid sometimes a sweat-soaked
dollar or less, to serve up paradise
on a bed of lettuce.
we college-degreed live
with our brains, the knowledge,
and the greed,
and pass the lettuce.

EARTH, SKY, AND PANCAKES

BY MARY HOWE

his morning I ate fresh strawberries and a buttered croissant in bed. The February sun reflected through the cloudless sky onto the sheets. A huge round blue porcelain mug filled with sweet coffee and milk in my hands, I drank and noticed that flakes from the croissant were clinging to my cream lace camisole. Breakfast felt extravagant and lush and warm. It didn't matter that I got crumbs everywhere because this was my pretend breakfast. None of it was real, except in the sense that what we wish for can be more defining than the physical world around us.

My real breakfast was frozen strawberries pulverized in the blender with unsweetened soymilk and protein powder. I drank it while standing barefoot on the kitchen tile looking out the window and wondering if I would get out to fill the bird feeder today. Almost unnoticed, a quarter moon asserted itself in the stark windswept sky. Breakfast felt cold, restrained, and sustaining. If I eat too many buttery French movie breakfasts, I get insecure and have to check out my ass in the mirror more often than I would prefer. This is part of the legacy of my past.

Certain formative experiences are with us always. They remain mysterious, but evolve as we do. They whisper what it is we want. Sometimes they tell us what to eat for breakfast.

◇ ◇ ◇

It started early. If you are an exuberant fat female child, life presents you with a good many arguments for why — although you might have felt magical and strong and glowing — really fat exuberant female children are not particularly appreciated in the American Midwest. They do not appear on Zoom or the Electric Company. They do not wave from parade floats. They are not the winners of talent contests. There is no power associated with the fat girl, other than, perhaps the power she can feel, her movement, her heartbeat, her feet on the floor. The objective power is the skinny woman in the mini skirt who is so important to flying that starship. It is the sleek, high-heeled beauty contest winners and the slender high school girls who get to drive their boyfriends' cars. The pretend self is invented. She is like me, but thin. She is like me, but a crew member on a starship.

Wishing won't get you there. By the time you are a teenager, you realize that you have got to develop sophisticated techniques. My friend Twink and I invented a rigorous discipline of reflective self-critique. This took place in front of any available mirror, but we did our best work before the big sliding panels of her dad's closet doors. You can't fully appreciate the innumerable unacceptable qualities of your body with just a cursory glance. You have to devote some time to the endeavor if you want to gain a deep appreciation. Yes, obviously my thighs are way out of bounds there – where they form an outrageous curve – but look closely at the inner thigh, there just above the knee... that should be concave. Now as we turn to the side, we see the line here where our ass meets our thighs is not what it should be. There should be a scoop there...the role call of overabundant flesh takes some time. You can't rush the process. Eventually we conclude the session and adjourn to the kitchen table to get high. Her dad's pot is lovely. Celestial green perfumed clusters with little white hairs that smell like seedless seventies heaven. What could be more ethereal than inhaling the confection of smoke, listening to Parliament Funkadelic connecting with the mothership, and reaffirming our values.

The importance of being thin: It is the good from which all other good must follow. There can be no good without it. We just want to be thin. That's all. We don't want to be rich. We don't want to be movie stars. We don't want boyfriends. We don't want a ton of clothes even. We would kill ourselves for being fat except for that improbable yet reoccurring optimism that thinness could be possible – and the horror of leaving behind a fat-assed corpse after shuffling off this mortal coil. The size of our want is greater than the size of ourselves, which, we agree, is ample. We are fierce.

Lying on a warm waterbed and watching cartoons with the sound off and Commander Cody and his Lost Planet Airmen on the hi-fi is wonderfully entertaining. You could just live like that forever if not for the insulin response from the pot driving your blood sugar so low that you are not what you could call hungry. Not really even starving. You are like animal hungry; like the slobbering coyote on the TV. You start to relate to the early Cro-Magnon who survived from smashing carrion bones with rocks and sucking the marrow through the splintered cracks. Bone hungry. The wolf is at the door and will not be turned away. Red-eyed, hell-bent for pork rinds is in profane opposition to the skinniness prime directive. But what can we do? The wolf is not going to go away. We have to cut some kind of deal. OK, what if we, just this once, make the tiniest batch of oh, say...pancakes and then, I swear – not eat anything at all tomorrow? I'm not kidding. Nothing tomorrow.

We are destined to eat pancakes. We did not choose our pancake destiny. There are circumstances that eclipse the best-laid plans; they are undeniable, like the force that moves the tides. When it is 4:38 in the afternoon and you are 14 and stoned and haven't eaten all day, the creation of a batch of pancakes is an event through which you can bear witness to the wonder of the universe. The perfect little bubbles rise then pop, leaving the air vent tube and signaling the spatula wielder that it is time to flip the miraculous batter circle over. It is a cake...but simple, primitive. You might find something like this cooked over an open fire in Uruguay, or Ethiopia. Women cooking cake. Our cake is primitive, but it has the same soul as the *éclair* and the *petit four* that the pig suede-heeled women in Paris lust for. The pancake is the simple soul of cake. It is the most lovely, feminine, round, sweet, soft, forgiving matter in the Milky Way. Round like a breast, round like an egg, round like the moon. In celebration of the abundance you twist the cap off of Mrs. Butterworth's head and out pours sweetness. It pours right out of the body of the woman; right out of the top of her head. Getting to eat those pancakes is unimaginable good fortune. Like finding a vein of gold on the dirt. There is no choice here, anyway. Not eating the pancakes would be like not breathing. We become one with the pancakes and have three big glasses of milk. The cake is earthly, grounding, bringing us back home. Home. Home, where the mirrors are.

We don't even say anything. Do not pick up the sticky dishes. We leave Mrs. Butterworth with the top of her head open and make the dreadful passage to the sliding mirror doors in the bedroom. Now we must pay the price. Frightened to look but perversely driven to do so, we take in what lies before us. It is impossible to imagine that those are our bodies. We are separate from the people staring back at us. There is nothing wrong with our body image. We feel perfect. We imagine that our bodies are the tight, lean, model-thin figures that represent female power. Real power. Undeniable sway. We feel it. We know when we emerge from the ocean of our being that the drops of sea water will roll off beautifully defined, concave inner thigh muscles. We see the rippling cuts in our shoulders, the achingly beautiful curve that defines our waists. We *feel* it. We know that that is who we are but... What the fuck is this in the mirror? There is just fuzzy, round dullness. We are drones, drudges. Stringy hair, overly round cheeks, oily skin, Oh no no no no no no no no. Tight pants! Awful tight pants. They are a size larger than the ones we would like to wear, anyway. They cut into our crotches and make obscene bulges where our labia are smashed against the fabric. The guys call girls like us "crusty," meaning disgusting, like dried scabs on a sore. Somehow the fat makes you dirty. Undesirable, dirty, powerless.

When you feel like hell's own whale and are more miserable every minute you stare into the sliding glass mirror, one thing is certain. You must not abandon the project. This might, for instance, be a good time to try on some clothes! Maybe this whole phenomenon with the light being reflected off the mirror and absorbed by the cones in our eyes is a huge mix up! Could there be some mistake? What if really we have lost weight? A scientific investigation must be undertaken to test the theory. We will take subject A: stoned 14-year-old girl who has just consumed a pound and a half of pancakes and three glasses of milk and see if said subject can fit into the stimulus B: a pair of pants previously thought to be far, far too small (so small that they were given to friend who might be slightly less unlikely to gain entrance.) *If* subject A can get into stimulus B, then we will conclude that previous correlations between subject's appearance and what we know to be "crusty" were erroneous.

So you take off the larger pants, the ones you were wearing which were undeniably too tight, and you step into the much smaller pants. Just getting them up to your knees is an accomplishment. It is immediately apparent that there is no way these pants are going on. OK, we have to admit right off that we will not be able to wear these pants, not even just to the 7-11 to buy some cigarettes. Still...if we could just get them on and buttoned, that would be something.

Denim will give a little, and flesh is malleable. Through the use of excessive force, which actually causes a belt loop to tear off, we get the pants up to our crotch. The zipper splays open at 180 degrees. Success seems unlikely, and even if it can be achieved will really only serve to prove a kind of stubborn insanity, but giving up is too heartbreaking. Having already been defeated by a plate of pancakes, it is unthinkable to succumb also to a pair of size 7 pants. Exhale, suck in, curl torso forward, pull the sides of the zipper together.... Tug the thing up. Shit. The zipper catches some of that bulging flesh. The skin actually gets zipped in. That really hurts. Ouch ouch ouch ouch. Unzipping it hurts, too. Try again. Faster this time. Now the button. OK. Goal attained. Now let's enjoy the event. The sausage skin fit creates a rippling cascade of fat rolls over the top of the pants. Butt and thighs have merged into a single squashed entity. Walking is out of the question but a sort of pivot ambulation is possible so that the spectacle can be viewed from all angles. Well, even a hollow victory is a victory.

Removing the pants is easier than getting them on but still trying, like descending the summit of a mountain after a tough climb. Pants shed, quantities of tiny blood blisters in horizontal lines are visible on my upper thighs. The broken skin on my stomach is bleeding a little. I put the old pants on and they feel ultra loose and relaxed. We go back to the kitchen table and sit at the other side, away from the sticky dishes and roll another joint.

✧ ✧ ✧

That was 25 years ago. Getting high is out of the question now and I certainly don't eat pancakes, though I sometimes feel their gravitational pull. People don't get it. "You're so thin." Yeah, I know. But I once suffered a brutal attack by a pair of size 7 pants. "Oh my God! What happened? Did they catch the pants? Did they lock them away?" No. They are still out there. I don't think they can hurt me again, though. I am ready for them now. My want is no longer bigger than who I am, and I eat the breakfast that is whispered to me by the quiet voice that knows what I most want.

FORMS OF THE DISEASE

BY ANNA HUSAIN

Seeds, skin, pulp, flesh, pointless
Regurgitate the sickly sweet insistence
To eat and be something
To hold and admire
While becoming less
Yourself

Is a pound worth so much
Inching up or down the scale
Tallied, judged, swallowed, revisited
Oh, to be weightless, ethereal
Invisible
To conquer hunger's realities
To hover lightly above the earth.

PREPARATIONS

BY ANNA HUSAIN

With my hands, I recreate his world,
the world he left behind, a country
of spices, the scent permeating
mortared walls of domiciles, grease splatters, a history
of meals, the happy sounds of kettles, their spouts
forever singing hospitality.

I know he misses them.

With my hands, I chop and mince memories,
onion, tomato, garlic, ginger, they intermingle
wife and mother, two cultures, one teaching the other
shared recipes, passed down through generations,
measuring years in generous handfuls,
the presence of family behind each mouthful.

I know the price of forgetting.

Chutney, kabobs, curry, I have learned them by heart
from the woman who bore him, my cupboards filled
with strange herbs, now familiar, his stories
of childhood hunger, forever connected to the life
of my kitchen in America.

I know he is weary

of years, set apart, so his appetite cries out
for a taste of identity, what is left, what is never again to be, the boy,
feeding at his mother's table, she
growing the man I will one day marry.

He is well fed, Amma, he is well fed.

TAKE TWO?

BY SALLY JONES

y old voice surfaces every now and then and says, "Is there really such thing as taking two of anything, especially food?" If I was inclined to eat two, it generally meant that I enjoyed it enough to leap towards the place of "more." I used to define "more" as anything beyond the number two.

My long-standing relationship with bulimia supports that two is an illusion. One is never enough; two hundred is too few. I would allow myself one of any morsel of food in front of others, but if I felt the desire for more, my psyche was nudged into social etiquette and I began to behave in coy ways to feed the hunger.

I was numerically challenged. I spent most of my life counting calories so that the numbers on the scale would drop. Losing one pound was never good enough, losing two never happened, and losing more was always a good reason to celebrate by going shopping. I usually waited for clothing sales so that I could cash in on the bargains and save a dollar or more. My attention was always keenly focused on sizing labels. Anything beyond a six was not acceptable, so I would ditch garments of all other sizes and squeeze into something smaller just to fit into the social trend of desirable numbers.

If I dared to flirt with the ever illusive "two," I may have experienced a full-blown episode with my addiction during which I could scream from the depths of my being, "I am addicted to chocolate covered almonds, strawberry rhubarb pie, Godiva truffles with rich gooey toffee centers, Lays' BBQ potato chips, Beef Wellington, McDonalds' French fries, *escargots* dripping with lemon butter, and Krispy Kreme Doughnuts...." The list goes on and on.

I didn't need to hide in dark alleys with my "drug" of choice concealed in a brown paper bag. I could swoon openly with my love – without fear of being whisked away in a paddy wagon to a drug rehab.... Center. As long as the numbers all stayed in check, I could proudly stand in my size six jeans on any public property and howl out my words through a megaphone, if I so desired. Since most every person could relate to at least one food addiction, I may even have received applause for such a radical and brave declaration.

I could declare my love for food, but if I openly took "two" (or more) of anything in the presence of others and my size six jeans no longer looked comfortable, the megaphone would drop – whistling would turn to jeers, and the applause would slowly diminish. There I would stand, naked from the truth of my addiction, as a silent cloud of disgust would fall upon me from the crowd. I'd melt away with the remains of my last morsel of chocolate as the heat from my final words reflected on my bright red cheeks. Lady Godiva would make her presence known by drizzling down my face as shameful tears. I would then retreat to the safety of isolation where I'd secretly drink her away.

When confined in the solitude of my own guilt, I quickly found redemption through denial. I normalized my obsession, and eagerly awaited the next opportunity to indulge. My shyness for crowds led me to seek smaller, more informal gatherings like Sunday dinners with my relatives. I'd plan my life around the event to establish illusionary control over my passion.

If I were taken with a particular food at a family event, I would wait until nobody was looking and stuff more into my pockets. After I'd openly consumed a socially acceptable portion of food, I would assign myself to dish washing detail. It was the least I could do for devouring a lovely meal someone else had prepared for me. I would tell others to stay away from the kitchen and allow me to be the good little daughter that I am. So I retreated to the lair of my loved one, and made busy noises such as clattering of pots and pans until they gathered around to hear my father's latest story. Then I'd begin the dirty job of doing dishes while stuffing myself with the equivalent of three of four extra dinners.

Although I've always enjoyed feasting on a few favorite foods, I never committed to any particular one. I have always been an equal opportunity eater. I could easily betray a trusting relationship with Miss Vicki's Chips for a bucket of KFC. And Miss Vicki wouldn't care, either! She would always be waiting for me when I returned, drooling for that savory taste of sea salt. She'd never leave me; neither would The Colonel – not even for engaging in lengthy serial affairs with multiple foods.

Sometimes I could not find a reprieve from my guilt, and ripping the size 16 label off my jeans was no longer effective. I became stuck within the ugliness of cold, hard reality and felt an overwhelming sense of disgust with my unsightly affairs. I would look at my body and see remnants of every food partner I had dated. Fat ... Cellulite.... Stretch Marks, each taking the face of particular foods and laughing like demons for succeeding in taking over my body. Hurtful comments confirmed their ugliness and shame.

When "more" happened, so did the purge. I purged the dirty little demons until their faces no longer bulged and clung to my body. I purged until I acquired big lumps in my chest which I later discovered were my own ribs. I purged until more became negative two hundred. I purged my lust, my shame, and my guilt until I was dizzy and unable to walk or stay awake. I purged my body, heart and soul into total isolation. Only then, did I surrender to a higher power and fall into the arms of the earth-bound angels of E.D. Recovery.

To "detox" from an Eating Disorder, I had to follow a "normalized" meal plan (we never say diet because that infers deprivation). Nurses supervised meal times to ensure that every edible item on my plate was consumed. Lettuce became an instrument to wipe away all traces of salad dressing from its container. I was accompanied to the bathroom to deter an encore from the purge demon. I came into direct combat with the dreaded Number Two. Every cell in my body screamed, causing my stomach to rumble and process paired food items such as double-egged omelettes, two bowls of cereal, a pair of toast slices. This seismic activity pushed its way through my system as my body rebelled by belching, and expelling so much flatulence that a simple apology didn't come close to cutting it.

In my recovery, I did the math. I learned that society has been engaging in math abuse by using numbers to measure someone's self worth – and I have been enabling it. My E.D. Recovery Angels told me that fish are the only beings that need scales, so I threw mine away. I am now free from numerical definition and can nurture the seeds of every other aspect of myself that has lain dormant for so long. Through this, I cultivate a love for the deepest part of me rather than seeking a superficial infatuation through food.

I will always be a food addict, but it is impossible to abstain from my addiction. Unlike alcohol or drugs, I cannot give it up entirely. I now accept that loving food is OK, but finding love by losing myself in a smorgasbord is not.

With moderation as key, I've learned to stop counting and listen to the cues my body so frequently forgets. Sometimes, I feel that I am walking on a high, narrow beam with the abyss of too much on one side, and the mile-long drop of deprivation on the other. I'm convinced that the longer I walk this beam, the better I will get at finding balance between the two.

And so, I cannot entirely divorce food unless I choose to die. Neither can I experience or express love through overindulgence. Instead, I accept a formal "separation" from large quantities of food and strive to build a harmonious relationship within which I live in "matrimony" with a healthy balance of "more."

My journey to wellness has accelerated through numbers. I have realized that taking care of Number One is all about love. By learning to love myself, I foster a connection to my feelings, and the world. With every breath, my heart opens a little more. With the passing of every sunset, I learn the importance of truly living and loving life within the gift of my body.

MEATBALLS AND SPAGHETTI

BY LYDIA KANN

he couldn't cook for shit. Perhaps no time to learn, certainly she'd had no aproned mother kneading bread when she came home from school. One could imagine her stepmother making food for the two sisters along with her own daughter and sons, but surely she wouldn't have taken the time to teach the fine points to my mother.

I'd return home along 95th, past the two theaters on Broadway, maybe playing, "House on Haunted Hill," or a Judy Holiday hit. I'd stop at Johnny's Pizza for a slice – around the corner from the Thalia with all those foreign films so tedious with their little words along the bottom of the screen, favored by my mother's crowd, Eastern European immigrants who sure seemed quaint if not obsolete to· my 12-year-old mind. So embarrassing those short people; even the men often couldn't break 5'2". They'd cluster in living rooms at Brighton Beach and speak in tongues and sing or laugh with great gusto, certainly breaking my sound barrier. No shrinking violets there; they seemed to broadcast their foreignness, their otherness, their difference, as I shrunk, sunk into a fantasy of invisibility, and sat on the other side of the subway all the way home.

That mom of mine, no slouch in the observation department, would twist the knife of humiliation by playing up her oddness. One time coming home from the beach she sat across from me on the train, sensing my wish to not be associated with anyone so foreign and embarrassing. I pretended she was like any other strange passenger, and that I was there as an independent young adult, carefree, sophisticated, suave. When the train lurched out of Times Square my mother slowly tipped over onto the empty seats next to her, like a drunk, and watched my torment with a devilish smirk. I tried to stay disconnected from the scene, but when we got off my outrage was challenged by Mom's satisfied giggling. Real funny.

Anyway, on school days I turned down 95th and headed toward the park, past Amsterdam, where the ethnic vibes picked up, and halfway up to Columbus. Past the whispered invitations and loud taunts of "*Maricon,*" whatever that meant – it didn't sound friendly to me – past the looks from eyes of men in every color and build, and quickly into the lobby of number 150, the second of the only two real apartment buildings on the block. The rest were brownstones, short two story jobs that may have once been grand. They now were layered with children and adults speaking a mixture of languages, clothes hung out to dry, withered plants, neglected gardens, and occasional boarded windows. Number 150 and Janey's house next door stood tall, testaments to another history on that street. Maybe of less noise and less people, surely less color and energy.

I mounted the stairs. *Why didn't I take the elevator,* I wondered, and opened the door of 4C, a complicated maneuver of several locks and a deadbolt. What a way to live, with metal rods braced against the impinging world of evil outside, ready to beat down your door at any moment of vulnerability. A memory flash of the time my wallet disappeared somewhere or other, and a week later showed up through the slot in my apartment door, but why the slots? An image of my wallet, looking uninjured but missing the money it had held, dropped on the floor by the door through the slot of 4C. Some person, who was he, for sure a he, had found that empty wallet and read the ID and come all this way to drop it off up the stairs and through the slot in that door around the deadbolt and all the protective devices to land on the floor in my front hall. Go figure. Was he the evil thief feeling guilty or some Samaritan trying to balance out the scale of good and evil? I'll never know.

It must have been 3:30 by the time I entered the apartment on school days, and the light would be muted, through the dust on the windows and around the venetian blinds. I dropped my books – we carried them loose in our arms those days – and headed to the phone. Janey lived next door; well, actually our tall buildings were separated by a short squat house, but our important information was the possibility of seeing each other in our respective kitchens across the courtyard while we spoke on the phone. A complete Nancy Drew kind of communication. A sense of knowing but not really. I could see Janey, but only vaguely, and I couldn't tell what else went on in that apartment of hers. I knew her parents were working, but the rest of her life there was a mystery. They were Germans, even though Jewish, and still foreign. And that kind of foreign seemed forbidding, the accent a reminder of a dangerous, never to be spoken but always present, evil. I loved Janey, but it was sort of scary to go there. Her mom was tense or maybe just formal; her dad worked most of the time. Yet Janey and I could joke and laugh till milk squirted out our noses, and once when I was older I saw her nipple stick out under her training bra, and another time a cockroach was crawling around the button of her sweater. I never told her about either of those sightings, but they left a big impression.

Oh, I was talking about my mom's cooking, wasn't I? Well, after my phone call with Janey and homework and a sneak read of my latest novel from the library, my mother would make it home from work, from the factory on 26th where she sewed clothes and yakked with those ladies all wearing housecoats and big bellies and double chins. She would have stopped at the grocery and picked up some fresh vegetables; I always prayed they weren't limas which I hated the most, and maybe just peas in the pod and some string beans, a piece of meat or bread from the Babka. The meat spoke a story because it was usually lamb chops or filet mignon, and everyone knows you can't pay for fancy meat on a blue-collar salary. But I swear it was true, and it meant love or insanity − either way I can taste its bloody richness now.

Some days Mom made her idea of meatballs and spaghetti. She rolled small odd balls of straight ground sirloin and dropped them into a frying pan of bubbling Campbell's tomato soup. Even I knew that wasn't meatballs and spaghetti, but something about her effort to cook "American," although an Italian version, touched me, and I never cut through the bubble of our pretend. Sort of like Janey and the cockroach; some things you don't speak of, but they kind of make you cry.

PENNY CANDY SUNDAYS

BY ROXANNE KAZDA

We grew up the only Protestants on the block in an Italian Catholic neighborhood. Each and every Saturday afternoon Mom would give me a dollar, and I'd go with my sister Katy to buy milk at The Little Store down on the corner. Most neighborhoods had a corner store – some Italian, some Polish, but always smelling of sausages and cheeses and coffee and sweets. A dollar was a very big deal to us back then, because we knew that a gallon of milk cost 89 cents with tax, which meant we'd have 11 cents left over for penny candy. So off we cheerfully went, balancing along the curbs the whole way – that was the rule – to run our errand with the sweet reward at the end.

We pushed open the big heavy door, bells hanging from the handle ringing and clanging against the glass, and walked back to the cooler, filled with glass jugs of milk. The gallon was heavy for us, but thankfully, it had a plastic handle, which we took turns holding on the way home. We walked past the meat cooler displaying pastrami, prosciutto, head cheese and sometimes tongue, and reverently approached the counter by the big wall of penny candy. The choices were endless, and some were only two pieces for one penny, so we took our time and chose carefully.

Maria, the shop owner, was used to seeing us. We were there almost every day – for cheese, bread, sometimes for the little white paper cups of Italian lemonade, which was frozen and scooped in mounds into the squishable cup. At Maria's, you sure got your money's worth every day, but it was only on Saturday afternoons that we got to choose a whole sack full of candy.

Katy and I gazed attentively at the dizzying array of treats as Maria reached back around her thick waist to tug at her apron strings, and fastened a loose strand of wavy black hair up under her bun on the top of her head. Our concentration on the candy wavered for a moment since we were fascinated at her gold-rimmed teeth when she smiled. Sometimes she held a toothpick in between them, sort of as a hobby, which drew even more attention to the sparkle around the edges of her smiling mouth.

She reached for the small brown paper bag, snapping it open in a dramatic flourish as we made our decisions. So many choices: flying saucers, made of pastel wafers with little colored candy beads in the middle; red licorice record albums, with a dot of black licorice dead center; bull's eyes; Mary Janes; malted milk balls; non-pareils, with the white polka dots of sweetness on top; red candy lipstick, extra sticky in gold wrappers, to smear across our lips and feel all grown up; strips of white paper with dots of color pasted on, to be bitten off with our teeth, bits of paper also swallowed; and little wax bottles filled with colored sugar water, always a favorite, because after the bottles were emptied, the wax could be chewed for hours.

Maria was always patient and never hurried us in our choices - she knew how important these decisions were for us. This was a once-a-week reward, not to be taken lightly. Adults would be standing behind us, tapping their feet, drumming their fingers on the counter, but Maria was true to us, and never, ever rushed us. After we were finished, she sometimes threw in an extra piece for good luck, folded the little bag over at the top, just one perfect fold, rung up one dollar even on the big old cash register, the bell ringing out the finality of her sale.

We tried our best to hurry home, for the milk jug was heavy, the handle digging into the palms of our hands even though we took turns, and it became especially difficult to keep our balance on the top of the curb. But it was the rule, and there was no changing that. We also had to be sure not to step on any cracks, lest we break our mother's back, the thought of that responsibility heavier than the milk jug to our young minds.

Finally, we arrived home just in time for dinner, and we were each allowed to choose one piece of candy for our dessert. We chose the least favorite first, saving the best for Sunday morning Drive-in Church.

In summertime, after bath time and bedtime, we would awake on Sunday morning, excited and giddy about the prospect of Drive-in-Church. No need to change out of PJs, which was exciting in itself, and no need to wear shoes. A quick brush of teeth and hair, a bowl of Sunday morning bananas with milk and sugar sprinkled on top, my mom's checkered Thermos jug of coffee with yellow plastic cups steaming on the counter, and we were just about ready to go. The final – and most important – thing to pack for church-in-the-car was our precious bag of penny candy, which Mom and Dad always let us bring in order to keep us quiet and occupied.

Out the door, and into Mom's '49 Plymouth, light green, with gray houndstooth wool upholstery. Once there, Dad made his proclamation: "We're off," which he said every time we left for any place different or fun or unusual. Drive-in Church definitely fit into all categories.

Minutes later, we pulled into the big Harlem Avenue Theatre Drive-In parking lot, immediately recognizing other church members, all similarly attired. Dad found our usual parking place, six or seven rows south of the concession stand and dead center, just in case Katy or I needed a bathroom trip. We quickly rolled down the windows of the car while Dad hung the speaker on the glass and turned the dial to the right channel. We then looked up expectantly to the roof of the two-story concession stand, where choir members and the minister, my grandpa, were reverently climbing up onto the roof, silky red robes flapping in the breeze. Only the parishioners in our car knew the miraculousness of this feat, since we were the only ones that probably knew that Grandpa was deathly afraid of heights. That was surely a blessed event, getting Grandpa up onto any rooftop at all.

Older than my sister by just over a year, I tried not to show too much excitement as Katy wriggled from the thrill of it all.

Dad turned up the tinny volume in our window speaker, and we listened as recorded organ music began to play, the choral director's arms flapping in the wind as he feverishly directed the choir in theatrical solemnity. Grandpa stood in what the congregation saw as prayerful meditation, and what our family knew in reality to be stark fear. Hopefully, we were the only ones who noticed his white-knuckled grip on the edge of the pulpit.

When the song ended, we knew the long-awaited moment had at last arrived. Katy and I giggled in the back seat, our bare feet and legs tangled together in sisterly comfort as we carefully unfolded our little brown paper bag, sinking into the blessedly sweet morning.

THE SPIRIT OF THE RICE

BY MARIA LOGGIA-KEE

radition carries with it a sense of spirit. And obligation. Not everyone is set to inherit. The spirit passes from one soul to another, choosing and blessing. As the traditions are passed down from one to the next, it's as if the life of the past itself imbibes another. Nothing symbolizes this shared ancestry more than what goes on in my kitchen.

From an outsider's point of view, I alone stand at the counter, chopping up spices, forming breads, simmering onions on the burner. But in truth, I never cook alone.

Two days. That's how long it takes to make Easter Rice. I don't ever remember being shown how to make it, but somehow, sometime, I learned. The smells of cooking infuse the house just as the joys of cooking run through my veins. I may not remember how I picked up the patience, but I do recall when I had to take over the tradition. It was a few years after my great-grandmother, Nana, passed away.

My family came to California from Sicily via New York. I grew up with tales of making alcohol in the bathtub during prohibition. Bottles sold for a dollar. Nana went by another name – Diamond Lily. The Lily I knew was a true diamond, hoarded $20 bills in her support bra, recited the Rosary in Italian over me as I slept at night and constantly ordered, *"Mangia, mangia"* as soon as I entered the radius of the kitchen. Thick chunks of garlic dotted her hand-rolled meatballs. I used to pick them out, making a little pile of red-stained garlic on the side of my oval plate. Now, I roast the heads whole and spread the pungent paste on warm bread.

In her eighties, Nana, the matriarch, had held the family together. No one argued over Sunday meals of pasta and red table wine. After she died, Sunday dinners remained the same. Pizza rolled out on cookie pans continued to be made on Christmas Eve, but on Easter, baked mostaccioli took the place of the rice. For a few years, we lived without. Then I came of age. The age of cooking.

When it comes to Sicilian Easter Rice, the key ingredient is the sauce. Nana taught me the sauce recipe years ago. First, a blender purees the tomatoes. A stainless steel pot rests heavily on the stovetop. Small cans of tomato paste are opened, and spooned into the pot. Then comes the rest of the ingredients.

Nana stood in the kitchen in her worn flowered housedress, barely taller than me, and explained, "Two handfuls of salt, one handful of pepper." She transferred the salt poured into her hands into mine.

The measured amount filled over my cupped palm twice. The cold granules streamed through my fingers as the salt slid into the tomato mixture. My nose tingled as I blew the remaining pepper dust off my palms. Then came the magic of baking soda, which I later learned breaks down the acidity of the tomatoes. Only one-quarter teaspoon swirls and bubbles, making pinwheels in the sauce as it's stirred with a wooden spoon.

Fingers stained with the essence of garlic, thumbs dyed green from ripping apart basil leaves and throwing them into the pot. A small dollop of olive oil, but only if meat will not be added. If meatballs will be cooked, then the oils from the beef will keep the sauce from sticking to the sides. The sauce reaches to just below the rim. At the end of eight hours of simmering, it will condense down – thick and rich.

Nana's husband passed away long before I was born, his name given to my father. My grandparents' household consisted of my grandma, Papa and his mother, Nana. Fish on Fridays during Lent. Pasta every Sunday. Nana spoke Italish, a mixture of Italian and English. She would start a sentence in English, and change into Italian and sometimes back again, not always aware of what she was doing.

As proud as she was of her ancestry, Nana never wanted to return to Sicily. "Why look back," she would say. "We have a new home here."

◇ ◇ ◇

The eight hours that it takes to cook the sauce is not rest time. No. It's time to cook the meats. A chuck roast. A pork roast. An entire chicken. Ground beef.

Although it was never explained, I believe the reason so much meat goes into the rice is because of Lent. Not only was meat scarce in Sicily, but it is not allowed to be eaten during the Catholic Lent. The meat symbolizes the body of Christ. At the end of the forty days of fasting, in celebration of Christ's rebirth, comes Easter Rice, jam-packed with rich goodies.

The cooking of the meats is a slow, sensuous process. Succumbed in a baking dish, the chuck roast bakes in the oven. Since I don't have a double oven, the roasts are done one at a time. While the chuck roasts, the chicken goes in another oversized pot on the stove, and boils. Once the meat falls away from the bones, and the outer edges of the chuck start to brown, the two delicacies are finished. Then, they must cool before they are shredded.

The tender meat of the chuck roast falls into pieces in my hands. I could wait until it further cooled, but then the meat would not shred as easily. This way, the hot meat jumps from one hand to the next. I try not to scald my hands, as I quickly pull apart the pieces and place it in the orange ceramic bowl my grandmother gave me.

◇ ◇ ◇

My grandma came over from Italy during World War II. As a teenager, she lived in a convent outside of Rome. Once the war escalated, the nuns said they could not guarantee the safety of a budding 15-year-old woman. The soldiers already would break into their schoolrooms and urinate in the inkwells. The nuns feared worse would happen. Grandma was placed on a boat and shipped to America to live with relatives who had earlier fled. She grew thin from the journey and seasickness. Lice infested her long red curls. On Ellis Island, workers shaved her head. Even though her family could, no one spoke a word of Italian to her. Within one year, she spoke perfect English, without a hint of an Italian accent. And she was safe.

In America, Grandma held onto the superstitions of the old country. She couldn't give me a serrated bread knife unless I gave her a penny. If not, bad luck would fall upon me. As she grew older, her hands withered with arthritis. She knew the family recipes, but her will could not make her hands do the necessary work. As I stand in the kitchen, shredding the meat, I can feel her spirit through my body, with me, preparing the rice. Her once weak fingers, grasping mine and giving me the will to continue on. Feet sore. Hours into cooking. The tradition continues.

After I break the chuck apart, then comes the chicken. Tender meat slides off the bones; the skin goes into the trash can and the broth gets reserved for another meal. Wings are snapped open— every part must be used. I carefully remove the wishbone and rest it on top of the stove, near the oven vents, in order to dry. No one can say "no" to a little bit of luck. Luck is always wanted. Needed.

When I was in high school, Papa would trek across the desert on spring break, summer vacation and over the winter holiday. Vegas lay as an oasis; a gambler's dream. A promise of fortunes both known and unknown. Bathing in an oversized tub with my cousin in a suite at Caesar's Palace. Water gun battles at Circus Circus. The pink plush landscape at The Flamingo. Sun-heated pool at the Tropicana. While Papa slid silver dollars into the slots, I slid quarters into arcade games and dived beneath the soothing chlorinated water. One year, I got my ears pierced for the second time. Another trip, a third.

Papa is one of the reasons that I cook to this day. My living inspiration. With his wife and mother gone, he now looks to his oldest granddaughter to continue the tradition.

◇ ◇ ◇

Once both the chuck and chicken are shredded, I put the pork roast in the oven. Pork is not a meat that I eat often, especially in roast form, but there is something about the roasting during the holidays that transforms the meat into a delicious treat. After two and one-half-hours in the oven, it's usually ready to come out and cool. Throughout the entire process, the sauce must be stirred every half-hour. The wooden spoon is kept on the top of the pot, with the lid slightly askew. Every time I lift the lid to stir the sauce, condensation runs down the lid into the pot.

After the pork is shredded, added to the other meats and the sauce is cooked, everything goes into the refrigerator for the next day's preparation. On Easter Sunday, the ingredients all come together before going into the oven. Since dinner is more of a brunch and served at 2 PM, the day starts just after sunrise. Five pounds of rice are poured into a vat of boiling water. While the sauce reheats on the stove, the ground beef is broken apart and browned, drained and added to the other meats. Then comes the assembly.

◇ ◇ ◇

Although she was small in stature, Nana was strong. Cookies were made with 10 pounds of flour, enough spaghetti was made to feed a large extended family and all their friends. And five pounds of rice is more than enough to feed 20. A layer of rice goes into the baking pan, then the meats topped with sauce. My arm grows tired pushing the spoon, but never does the weight become too much, for there's always another pair of hands helping me, strengthening and pushing me along.

Before Nana died, she used to say, "If only I could see you graduate high school. That would make me so proud."

"You will," I'd say. "You'll be there. It's only a few months away."
She gave away all her jewelry in order to make sure everyone
got what she wanted. As she pressed her white gold and diamond
earrings into my hand, she said, "If only I could see you graduate."
And she did, from Heaven. She passed away one rainy night. I
was staying with her and Grandma while my parents and Papa were
away. A high-pitched wailing woke me, with Grandma screaming
my name.

"Call an ambulance. Please call an ambulance."

I called, and then followed them to the hospital. Too close in
order to see where the ambulance took them: my Nana, and
Grandma in the back holding her hand. Through red lights, rain
pounding against the windshield. Hours later, at the hospital I went
into the bathroom and noticed that my shirt was on backward, the
backings of the silver snaps reflected in the mirror. I didn't have the
energy to turn it right-side out.

I wore her diamond earrings to my graduation.

◇ ◇ ◇

Another layer of rice, meat and sauce is added to the pan.
Tears slide down my face into the *risotto*, the rice. The spoon grows
heavier with each subsequent layer. Cups of meat are mixed in,
adding to the richness of the meal. Once the pan is full, I put down the
spoon and smooth out the top with my hands, the rice warm, familiar.

◇ ◇ ◇

After Nana died my grandparents went to Sicily to see from
whence she came. She would never go back, but they would. When
they arrived, they opened a phone book, looked up their last name,
chose a long-distance relative out of the book and called.

"Our cousins from America are here," they said. "Come stay
with us."

And they did. Papa wanted to see where his father had been
born, a small city outside of Palermo, but the cousins would not
allow it. It wasn't safe. A death threat still lies against the family.
Some secrets do not die with the dead.

◇ ◇ ◇

Once the rice is ready, eggs are beaten and spread across the
top. The pan then goes into the oven, 350 degrees until the eggs are
cooked and the middle of the rice is warmed through.

Almost as important as the meal is the wine served with dinner. One year, six bottles of red table wine were consumed among eight adult drinkers. Papa always says that he cannot drink much because he'll be driving, but every year he has a few glasses.

At 15, Papa stole his older brother's birth certificate and enlisted in the military. Nana didn't know where her son was. One day, he waited during roll call and rather than calling out his brother's name — they called out his. With parental consent, the military let him stay enrolled. After that, Nana used to send him care packages of hollowed-out French bread stuffed with bottles of red wine. The wine helped him and his squadron buddies fight the loneliness of WW II.

After Nana died, we learned why she never wanted to return home. It was more than the fact that she had made a new home in America. It was more that she had left her own. When they visited our distant relatives, my grandparents got the full story, or a version of it. When great-grandfather was in Sicily, he got into a ferocious fight with another man. He killed him, and threw him down a well. The only way to be safe was to leave the country. And leave he did. First, he stopped at his fiancee's house to see if she wanted to flee with him. She wasn't home, but her younger sister said that she would accompany him to America. He was 25, and she was 15. And that was Nana. After she eloped with her older sister's fiancé, she never looked back. She always explained the lack of wedding pictures by saying that they had a small wedding. It was very small, indeed.

◇ ◇ ◇

Such a strong woman has ingrained such strong traditions. As the rice comes out of the oven, my father is ready to test. He takes a knife and cuts a hole in the middle of the pan, scoops out a mouthful and hums as his mouth closes around the rice. It's ready. The top gets smoothed back down. No puncture left in sight, and I place the pan on the dining room table.

Everyone gathers hands, and we bless the food on the table, and all that have come before. The spirits at rest for the time being, we settle down, and eat.

REMOVAL
BY AUSTIN KELLY

he mashed potatoes were lumpy. Just like her breast. With the careful skill of the finest sculptress, she held her fork by its end, and delicately modeled the pile of potatoes into two separate, adjacent mounds. Then she gently shaped each mountain's peak into a smaller, tiny bump.

She smiled, absently admiring the craftsmanship of her mashed potato breasts on the plate in front of her. They were amateur, certainly. This was her first sculpture. But then, it was also her first breast cancer.

The sick feeling welled into her gut for the thousandth time that day. She dropped the fork onto the plate with a clang, and bit her lip, holding back her tears. How many times a day for the rest of her life would that twist in her stomach slowly eat at her soul? How many meals would not be eaten because all she could think of was her breast?

Life sucks. Life is not fair. Life is a bitch. Life as you know it is over. What's the point of life anymore? The trembling voice in her head had repeated that again every time her abdomen cringed. She heard the voice now, as she stared at the uneaten steak and the glob of cream corn next to her lumpy potato breasts. It sounded desperate – as if her stomach were a towel, and someone was twirling it tight, then wringing it out. Unlike a towel, however, it wasn't water that flowed out. It was her spirit. It was her happiness. It was her freedom, and it poured out from her.

As the growing void, the emptiness that had encroached in her stomach, began to pass, she picked up the fork again.

She thought about cursing God. Someone told her, "God only gives us what He knows we are capable of handling." If God had only checked first, He might have given her a million dollars to handle instead. She was ready and capable of handling that.

Looking down at her breast, her right breast, she wondered where the left one was right now. What exactly does the hospital do with those things when they remove them? Throw them into giant plastic sacks marked *Defective?*

Should they do the same with her?

She remembered when the doctor had first said it: "I have to remove your breast."

"Take two," she'd responded. "They're small."

Turning the fork sideways, she scraped one of the breasts of potatoes off the plate, and onto the table. "Defective," she mumbled.

And then the voice again. *Life sucks. Life is not fair. Life is a bitch. Life as you know it is over. What's the point of life anymore?*

Angrily, she shoved the plate away from her and tossed the fork onto the table, finished.

It was hard to eat when you were being eaten. The food didn't taste right, anyway. Ever since she began the chemo, things tasted funny. There was a time when mashed potatoes were her favorite. Now they were just reminders.

She glared at the single potato breast still on the plate.

Modern art, she thought.

But then, what was she?

She certainly wasn't herself anymore. She was pale and scrawny: two things she never had been before cancer.

Then there was chemo. She certainly had hair before cancer.

It was as if she no longer thought of her life in the context of universal time. The Gregorian calendar was a stranger. For her, B.C. was Before Cancer. Everything later was A.C. That day, when she'd been told, had been the beginning of the end. Or at least, the beginning of everything changing.

A.C. life was life as a sick woman. A.C. was life as a dying woman.

People said, "You're not going to be a cancer victim. You're a cancer survivor." What the hell was that supposed to mean? Either way, she was still a cancer something. It was the cancer part that was the issue. Subsequent nouns really didn't matter.

Like the potatoes. Did it matter they were potato breasts? Couldn't she have made potato penises? Either way, they were still lumpy.

And either way, she was still bald.

Sometimes, to make light of it, she'd throw a lollipop in her mouth. Other times, she'd order, "You will order the finest gold chopsticks." Yet other times, she'd point and command, "Make it so."

Make it so was her favorite. Her daughter liked that one.

Her daughter. She wanted to see her daughter marry. She wanted to spend time with her mother. She wanted to be with her husband.

And then she realized the answer to the question she'd been mulling the entire A.C. portion of her life.

The point wasn't that life is not fair. The point wasn't that life is a bitch. The point wasn't that life as you know it is over. The point was...

She reached out, pulling the plate towards her. She picked up the fork, and scooped a large section of the potato breast into her mouth.

The point was living.

THE UNEXPECTED

BY WILFRID R. KOPONEN

I was bedecked with flowers, frills, and furbelows for what was meant to be – and what the Old Thing thought would be – a blissful, felicitous day, the day on which comedies traditionally draw to a close, ending with "and they lived happily ever after" or some other literary equivalent, even simply "The End" (until that also became old-fashioned). But no, the book in which I appear does not even open until decades after that day, and it was most decidedly not a joyous one, even though, I am glad to say, I was spared the knife.

Year after year, millions of high school freshmen become acquainted with me, quite against their will, I'm afraid. If I still have the power to move them at all, I elicit perhaps a chuckle or two. The sentimentality of my day and age has gone quite out of fashion, from what I can tell when the book in which I am interred is opened, and I observe the passing parade of fashion, along with the tedium, peer pressure, and raging hormones (as you would say nowadays) that are the signature traits of the high school student. Even if students' snickers indicate how pathetic I appear to those who meet me, generation after generation, perhaps it should be some comfort to me that I have not been entirely forgotten.

Some of my cousins (I speak metaphorically, you must understand), though they were queens for a day in their finery, have long been forgotten, as those who made their acquaintance have themselves passed from this vale of tears and are now in greener pastures. (In my day, people actually used such phrases seriously, however incomprehensible that may seem to you.) Others of my cousins were more fortunate, perhaps, being preserved in the photographs that were still a novelty when I made my novel appearance. (Pardon my little play on words; I have little to amuse myself in my dreary existence.)

Some of my cousins have achieved a different form of afterlife. After their demise, they were carved up — or rather, what was left of them was carved up — and preserved for posterity, immured in little be-ribboned boxes. (What people do to us really takes the cake.) I believe that some of you still follow this sentimental Victorian custom, although perhaps its popularity has waned since its heyday, when I was a sweet young thing. In its own way, this manner of preservation is analogous to the medieval custom of placing pieces of saints' limbs in reliquaries to inspire religious fervor. But even religious devotion is subject to the whims of fashion (as I have learned through the years), and in my day, the locus of devotion had shifted from the chapel to the home. Martyrs had been replaced by wives and mothers as objects of pious devotion.

The white boxes that house relics of my cousins have little in common with the bejeweled reliquaries of a bygone era, unless marriage itself is a form of martyrdom, a thought that your more cynical age might entertain. The Old Thing (as I think of her) traipses around these musty rooms in her yellowed gown. Ask her whether she agrees that marriage is a form of martyrdom. Ha, ha! I have grown bitter, as she has, in old age. Surely she would say that her form of martyrdom is far worse than the martyrdom of even the most unfortunate devoted wife, and no sorrow is like unto her sorrow.

The Old Thing and I have grown bitter, but I used to be delectable and sweet! But now, things vile and rank possess me merely. All right. If you must know, I have to make my own jokes, even if they may strike you as half-baked. Do you think the Old Thing would crack any? She's what you, dear reader, would in your time — although the expression was unknown in my day — refer to as a Drama Queen. So I think of the Great Dane, another author, another century, and another literary genre entirely, to distract me from my own grotesque role in the novel in which I live, move, and have my being. (Again, I speak metaphorically, as I have what could be called a sedentary existence.) But the Dane's lines could just as well have been uttered about me. Would that anyone were possessed of the wherewithal to listen to my lamentations! Alas, my rest is silence.

Yes, I may be pathetic in my decrepitude, but so too is the Old Thing. Yet neither she nor I have always been this way, although you, dear reader, became acquainted with us when we were already long past our prime. You must believe me when I tell you that like her, I too was once dressed in white and possessed of shapely curves.

I was all tarted up; the layered look never goes out of fashion. So was she, for what she, at least, thought would be a joyous occasion, although I was admittedly a bit more ambivalent, as I've always had a phobia about sharp blades. In hindsight, I now recognize the irony of this fear, for I have lived to a ripe old age (an overripe, ancient age), and, unlike my cousins, no one has ever jabbed me with a knife or cut me to pieces.

But back to the joyous day. The Old Thing and I were not the only ones here then. When people entered the room in which I was the centerpiece, I had the power to turn heads; I was quite a looker, if I do say so myself. But what good does it do to dwell on the remembrance of things past?

All you have as testimonial to my erstwhile beauty is my own words. You only see us as the pipsqueak and Star see us. Well, the Old Thing doesn't exactly call the girl Star; the Old Thing uses the Italian word (or maybe the Latin word; I'm not quite sure). I'm English, and English is the only language I know (other than the language of love), so the English word is good enough for me. Yes, by the time Pip, Estella, and you first glimpsed us, the Old Thing and I were not much to look at – except in horror and revulsion. Even the spiders that now dwell with me crawl over me without giving me a second glance. How the mighty have fallen and sunken!

Charles Dickens, as I did, eventually became more than a little bitter. Why else would he have called his novel *Great Expectations?* The Old Thing – you know her as Miss Havisham – was jilted at the altar, while I remain, no doubt, the most debased example of the culinary arts in all of English literature: her wedding cake.

MEAT

BY KATHERYN KROTZER LABORDE

e's all cowboy swagger and almond eyes, long legs and dusky skin, and I'm in his arms once again, though the moment is over in a burst of bright, powdery colors that scatter and settle across the desert.

It is a dream, after all.

And I want so badly for this moment to last, but time and again it is all so slowly sucked away from me – his face, this dream, my happiness – as he opens his mouth to speak.

I want to say the dreams started when I finally realized that I had to be, no-way-around-it, missed-periods-and-blue-plus-signs-don't-lie pregnant with Mu Bob's baby. Pregnant with a baby from a singing, songwriting, swaggering cowboy wannabe who was God knows where – maybe still in New Orleans? Maybe gone back to Texas? Me, pregnant, and no longer in New Orleans. In Berkeley. With a woman. With Sally. This has happened so fast.

The dream was always the same: me and Mu Bob Yang, in the desert. Sex in the sand. The imagined taste of metal, a strange tasting meat. A gun goes off. I return to this dream over and over, picking up new details here and there. But no matter where I enter the dream, I know where I am. I am in his arms as I was all those times. I am with him in the desert, as I was with Sally that first time she kissed me. And at that moment, in his arms, I am happy. I am home.

When I wake up, my skin is covered with sweat. I wonder if I've made noises. I feel cold and reach for the quilt and quietly, quietly drag it over my body. Sally Starsong is a solid, shallow-breathing shadow next to me, more real than the seedling afloat in my belly.

Sally loves me. Loves me in big ways – flowers on the table, oil-and-bubble baths drawn and waiting. She fixes dinner night after night – chicken from the whole food store, snap beans from the Safeway – and makes me take bites of everything. I can't hold it down. She follows me to the bathroom and hands me a moist, warm wash rag. She rubs my back and tells me in a low, happy voice how she'll always be there for me and the baby, how everything will fit so perfectly into place. Most times I believe her – she is wonderful to me – but then I have that dream, and I remember.

◇ ◇ ◇

He's in me and it's wonderful. Though the sand is warm beneath me I feel I am floating. A cool, full, watery feeling spreads and relaxes my hips and I want to hold it there forever. I say something to Mu Bob about love or want or need, something. I search his face for clues, but his eyes are dark under the Stetson's rim, and his words are lost in a rush of sand on wind.

Across her left hip is a fresh tattoo of a star eclipsing a moon that's quartered and blue as ice against the milky stretch of skin. Starsong and Luna, Sally and me. Some nights she visits this new coupling with her fingers, skating over and over the spot till she relaxes into sleep. Other nights she places my hand there. She is quiet when I touch her, rocking against me all the while. I am learning to use my hands, to master the reciprocal mystery of sex with a woman. I do as I would have done to me, all the while imagining the response, the inescapable trembling, so that I forget somehow that it's her body and not my own.

Sometimes I imagine the sand and the warm wind when we are together. I close my eyes and see a cactus standing tall against a Technicolor blue sky.

◇ ◇ ◇

Picnic. Drive to the Pacific. The trees pass by in a dizzying rush I try to ignore. Sally has packed baked chicken breasts and strawberry tea.

She talks of consignment shop cribs and flea market finds. Should we move? Should we stay? It is too much, I want to say. Actually, I want to scream. Maybe we moved too soon into an apartment, a relationship, a life, but I say nothing. I want to say that maybe this was just a rebound sort of thing for her, well, for me too, but again, I say nothing.

"I was thinking," she says, "about her name."

To name it would be to make it real, to make it more than just "it." I wish for a nap at that moment. But if I take a nap I'd wake up and feel like a truck had run me over. Napping is all I want – I am so tired – but napping kills me. There is no winning.

Sally tilts her head the way she does when she's thinking. "I think we could go with a moon theme. To go with Luna."

I look out the window. "Theme?" I have nothing to say that would be nice.

"Soooo..... how about Gibbous? Gibbous Luna."

"Gib-us? As in, 'Gib-us oh lord, our daily bread?'"

"It's a moon phase," she says. "Gibbous."

"Too hard. Too weird. No one will ever know how to say her name. Or spell it. People would call her Gibby."

"Unless she's a boy."

"A boy?"

"J-O-N. Jon. W-A-N-E. Wane, like the moon phase."

"Jon Wane Luna?"

"Jon Wane Luna."

She beats the steering wheel. She laughs and shakes her head. Saddened, I think of my dream; nauseated, I taste metal. I roll down the window, let the hard, cold air press my eyes shut, and wait for the feeling to pass.

◇ ◇ ◇

His words hit my ears in murky echoes of a language assumed rather than heard. It is the language of dreams, but I don't understand. Instead, I am moved by how beautifully the tumbleweed bounces along the desert floor, and how strong and green the cactus stands against the harsh blue sky. Looking at the cactus I think I'll never be as happy as I am right now. And it's not until I hear her voice that I turn back to face Mu Bob.

"I wanna teach her to swim," she's saying. "So she won't be afraid like I was. I wanna put her in Karate classes, or maybe Tae Kwon Do. So Gibbous can kick the shit outta anyone who picks on her."

At this moment the baby is nothing more to me than a metallic taste in my mouth, than a state of nausea and fretful exhaustion, than an invader lodged and growing in my belly. I cannot imagine the thing having a gender, a face, a life.

"I wanna take her hunting," she says. It was a strange thing to hear, since I didn't know she hunted. Even stranger to hear her say it while she pushes her hands into the dough. Bread, for dinner. "Some of the best times I ever had with my daddy was in the blind on those cold, cold mornings, waiting for the ducks, drinking coffee from a Thermos. It was so peaceful."

"Not so peaceful for the ducks."

"Well, if you've got a problem with it, we need to talk about it. We need to make some decisions here."

"We? I think you've just decided to teach her to hunt."

"It'll teach her to be self sufficient. To be responsible," she says.

"Responsible for what?"

"Responsible for what you kill. Do it the right way. Eat what you kill. Hey, survival skills wouldn't exactly be bad for her, you know."

Her eyes are on me; I can't look at her. I watch her hands pulling and patting the dough into two mounds. She tosses the mounds into oiled loaf pans. She places the pans on the windowsill and covers them with dish towels. She shakes her head as she walks to the sink.

"OK, then," she says, washing her hands. "*You've* gotta start thinking about these things. How *you're* gonna raise her. What *you're* gonna call her. What *you're* gonna tell her about me."

I leave the room. I know she is right, that I should be thinking ahead, but I am too exhausted to see past the weekend. Sally, on the other hand, has it all planned down to the gender, but I am coming to realize that is just the way she is. Sally acts immediately. She falls in love and gets a tattoo; she dreams up names for a fetus not in her body. She looks the world in the face and changes that world to suit her. She kills, then eats what she kills. Life is earth and sky, with no fog rising from the water to obscure the horizon. There is only day and night, with dusk but a momentary hindrance.

She tells me over and over that I am letting my life happen to me, but I am quick to point out that I am letting a life happen *in* me, which is something I never planned on, and something she can only imagine.

◇ ◇ ◇

His words may be lost to me, but Sally has no trouble hearing him. She walks past us, not looking at me and glaring at him. The rifle casts a shadow in the sand as it rests on her shoulder. I find myself reaching out to take it. I imagine tasting it. I imagine it going off.

Doors and drawers open and close as I pull up a kitchen stool to watch her, amazed as usual by how easily she uses her hands. She lifts the chicken and pats it, rubbing oil into the pink skin and powdering it all over with rosemary and sage, humming all the while.

I turn away as she stuffs it with fruit.

The days are passing. I catch myself staring at walls and out of windows, imagining conversations with Mu Bob that never took place and will never occur. I take my vitamins — sometimes they stay down. The last thing I want to do is to eat, but the doctor says I've got to try, that I've got to take control and think about the baby. That I don't want to end up in a hospital connected to a tube, fed without effort on my part, floating through the hours in a darkened room.

◇ ◇ ◇

From the corner of my eye I see an iguana scampering toward us. I can't move, can't speak. Sally is talking to Mu Bob in the dream language and I can't understand a word. I want to say something but all I can do is watch. Wait. And in a moment it's all over.

I look forward to bedtime; sometimes it's all I can think of, that time when the cool expanse of sheets is all mine, for a while at least, while Sally watches television in the other room. I try to remember every detail, not of the dream, but of my weeks with him. Sometimes I think I can feel him, catch the tide of his breath along my neck. At other times I think I can see how his face looked in the street light that first time he kissed me. Sometimes I see him as he was, and other times I can see the two of us there, me a rag doll in his arms, and I hear the soft undercurrent of his breath. I repeat the moment over and over, try to see through the gin-and-tonic haze of that evening to what it was that brought us together, to the moment where he pulled me to his side and walked me to his car.

Other nights I can't help but see how he looked out the window as he told me I'd be better off without him. I pulled myself away from him, thinking he'd stop me in the middle of the night. But of course, he didn't.

◇ ◇ ◇

The rifle falls to the ground and Sally reaches over to get it. "Nice shot," she laughs. "Not bad." She twirls it around like a baton. Thinking of it now I have to smile, she looks so funny, but it's not so funny then. I find myself watching the rifle. When I look around I see that Mu Bob is gone. I crumple to the ground and for some reason reach for the iguana. His body is warm in the sun. I squeeze the wrap of his skin and pull out a piece of meat. "Don't eat that," she tells me. "It's nasty."

It tastes familiar in a way I can't explain, and somehow bitter.
I spit it out, look up and see Sally smiling at me.

And then she says it: "There are worse things than settling – "
then her voice is garbled in that language that eludes me and I don't
understand until she says "someone who loves you."

There are worse things than settling down with someone who
loves you.

There are worse things than settling for someone who loves you.

There are worse things.

When Sally kissed me that first time I should have been
thinking about her. Instead, I was remembering Mu Bob's shoulders
against the midnight backlight of the open bedroom window, and
how I finally got out of the bed and sat in his lap, wrapping myself
around him that last time. I breathed him in. I told him I loved him.
I told him I wanted him to come back to bed. I made myself very
small and pressed into him to make myself one with him. I pressed
my wet cheek against his and told him that when we looked into
each other's eyes, when we sat on his porch, when he played his
guitar, when he sang to me, when we kissed, I wanted so much more
than just sex. I wanted late night rounds of Scrabble, and I wanted
sweet Sunday mornings lazing over coffee and newspapers, and I
wanted laughing with the lights out, and I wanted holding hands as
we walked to the corner store. I wanted conversations that lasted
for years.

He didn't hold me. He didn't move. But he spoke. And it was
only when I remembered what he said that night as I held on,
shivering with grief, it was only when I remembered those words
that I was able to give in to Sally's arms, to let myself be lowered
onto the warm white sand, and to wonder at the way she smiled as
she whispered my name.

◇ ◇ ◇

I keep my dream to myself, dipping into it again and again as
though it were a hidden box of chocolates. When I wake, my heart is
a stone, and my head literally buzzes with something far more
pathetic than what I still feel for Mu Bob, or what Sally says she
feels for me.

Sally Starsong, if it weren't for all those damned baked chickens I'd probably never eat at all. I would lie here in the dark until I was floating halfway between my dream and the reality of the bed I've made. Just floating and starving until, finally, my body would turn on what is sucking the life out of it, for nourishment. Slowly and silently killing before somberly and responsibly eating.

THE DIET

BY C. J. LAITY

Snack it, chew it,
      not another pound there
      burn it away sleeping
          viral nightmare
Why does it feel so hollow
(Eat all you can swallow!)

Stuff it, shove it
      into the bloody machine
      past first-sign sores
          white tongue
Reach toward the gore
(And eat all you can swallow!)

Push it, drop it
      feverish body above it
      spoiled inside, alive
          cancellation date
A stain, raised like a flag
(Eating all it can swallow!)

Lose it, shrink it,
      is to be half-ghost
      give water to the pillow, over
          so-called sin
Be prepared, pneumonic end
(eat all you can swallow!)

BARBIE UNREQUITED

BY STEPHANIE JONES LAUREY

I gave my childhood to you, Barbie.
I unmatted your platinum locks
and sewed oil rags from the garage
together for your underwear. I gave
you modesty when you had none.

I could have made you drive
your plastic friends around
in an old Kleenex box, but I bought
you a Corvette, a moped, a whole
cavalry of Rapunzel-maned
horses. And what did you do for me?

The same year I folded you —
clad in your best gown and pumps —
into the corner of my hope chest,
I starved myself, lost 35
pounds in nine months trying
to be you. The nurses held
me in their arms, carried
me from dinner chair to bed,
changed my clothes, and combed
my bleach-blonde hair.

I don't hate you for being thin,
Barbie, or beautiful or even too good
for food and sex. It's your smile
that haunts me — heart-shaped
and constant, an old lover's
valentine I can't throw away.

PICKLE DAYS

BY MICHEL MAGEE

Scalded wide mouth Ball jars
Suck sunlight from kitchen windows,
Ready for cucumbers
Still hugging earth,
Entwined on pole and fence
Inside the garden gate.

My arms and bare legs itch
From daily harvests,
Prickly vines reluctant
To yield nights' tangled labor
Of dew-diamond newborns.
I twist and tug, victorious,
Baskets heaving near noon.

By five the house is ripe
With vinegar's punch to the nose,
Onions' gouge to the eye.
Salt and errant mustard seeds
Litter the counter, turmeric stains
The chipped enamel kettle and
Fingers ache from ice and slicing.

TOO MANY COOKIES?

BY MICHEL MAGEE

Soup drips
on my new sweater,

no chance at hitting the napkin
spread across my lap.

My bosom, once small hillocks,
has shifted at glacial speed like

an unmoored continental plate
toward a wasted waist.

Was it too many cookies,
or simply mid-life's rearrangement

of a once heavenly body,
now foreign as the moon?

Someone pass the Oreos, please,
to pepper my sweater tweed.

IN RESTAURANTS

BY PAMELA MALONE

am six years old and in a department store in Cleveland with a stranger. I have been told she is my great aunt. All I know is that she looks like Little Lulu's mother and was eager to take me on this outing. I am visiting from California, and there is nothing particularly exciting to me about this dark, dusty store. But she has taken me first to the toy section and bought me something wonderful. A silver baton. This is the kind of extravagant luxury I could never hope for in my everyday life and I am spellbound staring at the bright silver shine in the dim light.

And now we are down in the lunchroom. A table with a Formica top, and this kind lady is eager to talk to me and ask me questions, as if what went on in my already cluttered six-year-old head were really important.

And then the waitress appears. She is pretty in a starched apron and matching white cap on her head.

My great aunt orders whatever for herself and then says with a smile, "She'll have the children's special lunch."

And I am asked whether I would like peanut butter, tuna or cheese, and I say, "peanut butter," expecting just that.

The waitress appears again with a chest of drawers, almost small enough to fit in a dollhouse. Out of the top drawer she takes a little red checkered table cloth about three inches square which she puts in front of me. And then from another drawer comes a little china plate with a flower on it. And from another, a tiny china cup. It is all so cute, and I find myself turning like Alice into someone very tiny, as I eat my miniature lunch, a little finger sandwich with no crusts, a thimble full of mashed potatoes, and one carrot cut like a rose. I am enchanted; so begins my restaurant life.

◇ ◇ ◇

Forty-nine years later, I am sitting with my mother in Bullock's tearoom. Only it isn't Bullock's anymore, having gone down the rung of the ladder from fancy chic to cut rate bargain. And my mother isn't my mother anymore either. She now has to walk with a cane, her fluffy white hair thinned to a few threads, her frowns from yesteryear gone. There is sweet acceptance in her face now, her voice so soft I have to lean forward to hear it.

She used to take me here when I was a teenager, and she'd tell me what I could and could not have. She picked my clothes, standing like a drill sergeant, repeating the mantra that I didn't look good in frilly things, "tailored suits you better," as well as the too oft repeated, "don't even look at that, it's too much." It was a continual battle of wills between my need to be me, and hers to count pennies and control. Somehow, a rabbit soft pastel dress that I would wear with pearls on my first college date, and a royal blue skirt and sweater set, snuck through.

This twice-yearly event was endured, but the swords were turned into plowshares as we rode the elevator to the top floor; the tearoom, where dreams could come true. My mother was never tight fisted when it came to food. Bullock's had a buffet, and we ate our delicate finger sandwiches, and pillow-like popovers with a shared ecstasy. The pot of Constant Comment was refilled, as we contemplated dessert, and the elegant models, sylphlike Audrey Hepburns, whirled before us in silks and furs.

Now the models are gone, and the buffet. But the light still comes in the window from some miraculous sky that is not the harsh and bright Los Angeles turquoise sky outside. The music is sweet, the waiter solicitous, and wonder of wonders, the popovers are the same. My mother and I are able to look into each other's eyes, the anger of the past gone, only love remaining. I lean forward and touch her silky hand, and say how glad I am to be back after such a long absence, and what a miracle it is, that in this city that continually destroys its past, this sweet place is still here, and so, again, are we.

◇ ◇ ◇

Women alone in restaurants observe intensely. The wine is red as a ruby, the waiter as handsome as a prince, the aroma of the soup, delicate enough to reach the soul. The waitress, who looks like a deer, brings my chicken tarragon with brioche; a poem forms, and I bend to write it down as Billy Holiday whisper-sings in my ear. I have been coming to this hidden place every year. A secret birthday present to myself. In this intimate interior, where flowers bloom in winter, I explore my mind's interior. The years pass, my sons have become men, the neighborhood has changed, and one bleak day I arrive to discover the restaurant itself has disappeared. But not those stilled moments when I lived in my own time, hovering like a butterfly over a flower.

◇ ◇ ◇

Women fall in love in restaurants. He told me the last one to finish the wine would marry first, and I saw the wine in his eyes, before our first kiss. And I did marry, but not him.

My husband and I fell in love over *wor won ton*, a rainbow universe of red, green and yellow vegetables, pink abalone, golden mushrooms and tangerine shrimp bearing gifts, silken doughy bundles that slid down our throats as we began that long swim through life together. We moved, our tastes changed, but still we are together, in restaurants.

◇ ◇ ◇

My granddaughter is six. We are sharing a glass dish of chocolate pudding topped with whipped cream. We take turns swirling the cream till it looks like a marble. The mirror on the wall reflects our faces as we dip our spoons in and look up at the blue ceiling painted with clouds. Those clouds, that whip cream, will last.

SLIPPERY

BY JOANNE MCFARLAND

Bold and bad
the way she wear
the scent they bake
their taboo stew
everything in it
cajun   overcooked

Badass to
sneak back home
sticky with his
paste
cooking dinner
like she ain't already
ate

Smooth Talking Man*

By Pamela Miller

Preheat oven to 350 degrees.
Prepare the following custard:
4 ounces ingratiating Frenchman
    1 cup Million Dollar Club salesman
    1 cup Luciano Pavarotti, firmly packed
    1 teaspoon Mephistopheles
Cook and stir in a double boiler over plenty of
hot water.

Sift before measuring:
    2 cups erotic poetry
Blend with:
    a 10-gallon hatful of honey
    3 barrels molasses

Beat well:
    1 wild, wild whirl around the
    dance floor
Add 1 forked tongue gradually. Blend until
thrilling. Beat in, one at a time:
    365 lies

Add the poetry-and-molasses mixture to the
lies-and-dance-floor mixture
in 3 parts, alternating with thirds of:
    1 quart extra-slick motor oil
    1 cup goose grease
    2 tablespoons mercury
    1 tube Brylcreem
Stir the batter until smooth-talking after each addition.
Stir in the Frenchman custard.

Whip until soft:
    1 patent leather tuxedo
Fold it lightly into the batter.

Bake in greased pan for about 25 minutes.
Cover, when cool, with:
    your body

*from *Recipes for the Perfect Man*

CUISINE Á LA COLEMAN

BY FRED MUHM

ull over, Pops!" Dennis' shout interrupted my thoughts; our morning hunt for deer had disappointed all three of us, with nothing to show for our efforts but bad tempers and sore feet. Though 16, his voice still rose to something like a shriek when he was excited, and he startled me, so I slammed on the brakes. For a few moments things were crazy; we whipped around all over the gravel road, and nearly rolled twice before sliding to a stop in front of a roadside stand selling game birds.

"Don't ever yell in my ear while I'm driving. Do you understand?" My sons looked sullen and got out of the car without so much as a nod. The boys soon returned walking side by side: Dennis, 5' 6 " and 180 pounds with his younger brother talking down at him from a skinny 5'9" – both curly-haired and shaggy. Allen carried a big, plump pheasant in full plumage, large as a super-size roasting chicken.

"Hey, Pops, here's supper." He clambered in followed by his brother and we drove to our campsite.

"I hope you guys have a receipt for the bird, 'cause we may just need it," I said, forcing my tired body from the car.

Dennis' mouth formed a thin, smug smile. "Don't worry, Old Man." He pulled the paper from his pocket, then shoved it back in as he carried his bow and arrows into the camper.

Allen had thoughtlessly – and typically – left the bird lying on the warm hood of the Toyota, so I grabbed it and began plucking the feathers from the gutted fowl and was half finished when I heard a grim voice behind me say, "You're in trouble, Mister; I heard you had an illegal bird here, and what I see confirms it." That scared me so much I jumped a good two feet into the air, spinning around and nearly losing my grip on our dinner. The game warden, all 6' 2" and 250 pounds of him, moved closer. "I'm placing you under arrest. Lean across the hood of your car, and place your hands behind your back."

"The bird is legal. We bought it from a game farm down the road, and my son has the receipt." I put the bird down on the table. He cuffed my right wrist, then snapped and tightened the other cuff on my left. It dug in painfully.

"Where's he now?" His face showed sweaty skepticism as he looked around.

"Inside, probably sleeping."

"Call him out here." He began to put the pheasant into an evidence bag.

"Dennis, come out here – now." No answer. Again: "Damn it, get out here now." Still there was no answer.

"Okay Mister, you're under arrest. Get into the squad car." His eyes were mere slits and the lips were a cruel, thin gash across the face. "Watch your head," he said as he pressed firmly on the back of it.

Just then, the door opened. Dennis, half-asleep with unfocused eyes said, "Whuz up, Pops?"

"Where's the damned receipt?"

"What receipt?" he said, still groggy. He rubbed his eyes, looking more like 12 than the 16-year-old that had been shaving off and on for a year; his disheveled curls partly covered his eyes.

"For the bird, birdbrain." I could feel the flush rising on my face, and knew I was losing control.

Dennis felt absently at his pockets, and mumbled, "Dun' no."

"Wake up damn it, or I'm going to jail."

Allan poked his head out the camper's door. "Here it is, Pops. Denny put it on the table."

The warden took the receipt from my son and read it. I watched the crimson migrate from his neck up. Then he thrust the slip of paper back at Allen, who took it.

"Sorry for the trouble, Mister," the big man mumbled, staring at his report form. "Gotta go see about this." He drove away in the dust, leaving another layer of dirt all over us.

He was barely out of sight when Dennis started in with his shit: "Almost, huh Pops?" He grinned, suddenly wide-awake.

"Shut your mouth," I shot back, still pissed about his slowness, and added, " No thanks to you – if your brother hadn't found that receipt, we'd have lost everything – car, camper, bows – all of it, confiscated."

"You were a trip – all scared and trussed up like some bad dude on the news that got himself busted, you know – for a bird!"

His dark eyes sparkled with delight at the image. "But no way, they can't really do that. Can they?" He seemed to like the idea.

I arched an eyebrow in his direction, "Care to bet on that? Good thing Allen had the receipt."

They went back inside the camper and reappeared with their archery gear. "We're going out again," Dennis said. "You coming?"

"Who's going to fix this pheasant if I do?" I could feel the sharp edge in my voice as much as hear it. "The least you two could do is help make dinner. After all, it's your idea. If it was up to me – "

"If we help you, we can't get any game. Can we?" Allen said. "By the way, we need the car keys." I took the keys from my pocket and threw them at him, hard. Startled by the violent action, he fumbled to catch them

As they drove off, I fumed to myself, *they're Nit-Wit and Half-Wit, with not a lick of sense between them.* "I finished plucking the bird and with a pair of pliers, viciously yanked pinfeathers. *Goddamned jackasses leave me with all the work; they'll pay for that.* I carried the bird into the camper and lit a camp stove burner. *I'd like to singe your asses.* I held the carcass over the flame, and turned it so that all the fine hairs were scorched from it. The pungent stench of burnt hair filled the confined space inside the camper, but the smell soon filtered out through the canvas walls.

My Coleman oven pre-heated over the burner as I rinsed the bird thoroughly, dried it with paper towels, seasoned it with salt, pepper, and herbs, and to add moisture, layered bacon inside and out. I slammed that dammed bird into an aluminum roasting pan, and the whole thing into a 350° oven; the food would be ready at five.

I mixed and cut baking powder biscuits, panned and covered them to prevent drying out while the bird roasted. I thought, *the two of you will regret leaving me with everything.*

◇ ◇ ◇

I reviewed the day's events: the dismal failure of this first morning's hunt and the warden's visit had stressed an already fragile relationship with my sons. They had pestered me until I'd agreed to take them on their first quest for deer – also the first time I had them both together since the divorce. I liked hunting, but with all the overtime at the plant, I had to take a week's vacation time just to get away – and try to settle these two unruly boys. Their mother said maybe some time with me would do them good, but in any case, she was done trying alone, and the time away from them could only do *her* good. I didn't like the circumstances one bit, and the boys were probably just as uneasy, but I couldn't know for sure – couldn't swear I even knew them any more.

My nose drew me back to the dinner.

◇ ◇ ◇

The camper's interior slowly filled with the aroma of the roasting bird, herbs, and the smell of freshly brewed coffee. The pheasant was done, so I took the roasting pan from the oven, and increased the temperature to 400°. Once I made some Stove Top dressing and put the biscuits in to bake, a couple of lengths of tin foil came in handy to cover the bird and dressing. *I should let it all get cold or eat it the damned stuff myself.* I mixed up some instant mashed potatoes and gravy and heated a can of corn so it would be all ready when the biscuits were done. *Maybe I won't let them eat or have any coffee. I need to have a talk with these guys, to set some rules for the three of us. They need to understand about sharing.*

They walked in just as I took the biscuits from the oven and turned the burners off. They inhaled deeply, grinned, and hurried to clean up for dinner while I opened canned cranberry sauce into a bowl.

My two freshly washed sons sat at the table, their wide-open eyes bright with anticipation. "Wow! Pops, it smells delicious. How'd you do this with just some cans and stuff," asked Dennis. He gestured with a sweep of his hand to show his appreciation – rare praise from him .

Allen cut in before I could reply. " Boy, I never knew you could cook so good, you know. Mom must have taught you, right?"

I just snorted and shook my head. "You can do a lot with food that's dried and canned, that's all, but I'm glad you appreciate my effort." *Equally rare praise.* "Let's eat before the food gets cold."

I prepared their plates, saying, "You don't deserve this." Each contained one tablespoon of potatoes and gravy, dressing, cranberry sauce, and one scrawny wing – all arranged to emphasize the scantiness of chow on the large platters. I watched for their reactions.

"What the hell is this," Dennis squawked. His eyes had grown to the size of silver dollars, and had it been possible his jaw would have struck the table. He sat staring at me, his hand poised in the act of reaching for a fork.

"Yeah, come on Pops, where the hell's our food?" Allen yelled. His face, initially shocked, was twisted with anger. I cut him off.

"If you two bird brains think I'm going to let you skate without helping around here, you're even crazier than I thought. You just got what you earned, and more," I said as I glared at him, my gaze meeting his, my body tensed. *This could get pretty sticky in a hurry; if one of them doesn't back down I may have to, and that would be disastrous. Damn it; this isn't what I wanted.*

Dennis recognized the danger signals and wisely said, "OK, we'll do the dishes and clean up. Just give us some food."

"And you," I asked Allen. My eyes locked on his.

"Yeah, yeah." His shoulders drooped and he looked away, adding, "You're one screwed-up, mean old dude."

Then I filled their plates with much larger portions of food. "After supper we're going to talk about showing respect for each other, and how things are going to be done from now on. Let's eat while it's warm."

The rest of the meal was finished with an occasional, "more bread here, or more..." The pheasant was perfect, with moist, succulent flesh that fell from the bones. The bacon's smoky flavor combined with the wild bird's was so good that my sons ripped the carcass in half and picked every shred of flesh and bacon from the body cavity; they had no trouble finishing the remaining biscuits, potatoes, gravy and cranberry sauce.

After the meal they started drifting towards their beds, halting only when I shouted, "Hold on! Remember what I said before dinner? Is this how you show respect for others? I busted my butt cooking that meal, and now it's your turn." I pushed back my chair and stood over them. "First, nobody freeloads here; we all do our share, and from now on we take turns doing the cooking and cleanup. Fair enough? If you can't cook that doesn't mean you can't learn, and if you can't live with some simple rules, you two can go home now," I told them. "Do you understand?"

"Alright. Give me the keys and we'll go home then." Dennis strained to bring his face within inches of mine, his hand held out demandingly.

"No! If you go I'll drive, and I know your mother will be upset when I tell her the reason you're home after only one day," I could feel the heat rising in my cheeks and my ears burning, and struggled to maintain my equilibrium.

"Bull! Why bring Mom into this? She hears you, she'll be, you know, on our case for days — no way." His bluster began to fade, and he backed down. "Oh, man," he whined, shaking his head. "Shit, man."

"My point exactly. We're pretty much stuck with each other, 'cause if you're taken home early, your mother's not going be real happy about this sudden change in plans — it's your choice," I said, relaxing as I saw his shift in attitude.

They cleaned up the mess, banging and clanging pots and pans around, and I thanked God for plastic plates and cups.

◇ ◇ ◇

The smell of freshly brewed coffee, burnt bacon and toast woke me the following morning. Dennis, looking a little more rumpled than usual, said, "I was making coffee and Screw-Up here burnt the toast; I was helping him scrape the burnt off when the bacon scorched and those — " He just nodded sadly towards a yellow mess in the pan, which spoke for itself.

Allen, who was pointedly ignoring his brother's insult, gave me the piece of toast with the least black around the edges, a glob of the springy, latex-like, scrambled stuff from the pan and a big heap of super crisp bacon. I tried to be gracious at their attempt to make things right. "Thanks guys, but why don't you have more on your plates?" They each had two slices of black toast, one slice of bacon and a small spoonful of eggs; I took my plate and redistributed the bacon and eggs equally among us. "Okay, eat up. We've got deer to hunt, and if things go right, we'll have venison steaks tonight." Manfully, we gulped it all down, helped by large swigs of strong coffee.

I got my buck that morning. We did have our steaks and a good day in many ways: that night the boys helped with dinner and learned about simmering vs. scorching, browning vs. charring, and taking out the garbage.

We all did the cleanup together.

THE DOCENT

BY CAROL A. MYERS

docent, Mama. It's a person who conducts tours, like in a museum. Oh, look, never mind. We'll be there in about 20 minutes," Alberto said. My son, the scientist, clearly annoyed with his Old World mother but barely able to contain his excitement. "Remember, now, they have more data than I could possibly imagine about our time and our society. What I want them to see – want you to show them – is how we *live*."

Of course. Why should this surprise me any more than anything Alberto has done since he was a child? Of course he understood time travel. Of course he had contacted another galaxy from the future. And of course he called to say he was about to bring three aliens home to his mother's house.

"And Mama?"

"Yes?"

"You don't have to feed them. I have no idea what they eat."

What kind of boy did I raise? Of course they would eat.

◇ ◇ ◇

If they were surprised to come in the back door, I couldn't tell. The back porch was jammed with pots of herbs, braids of garlic and plants of one sort or another rooting in colorful bottles balanced on the window sashes. Slender tendrils reached out to touch airy heads of dill. Sunlight bounced off the shiny surfaces of the mismatched plates serving as plant saucers as well as the bald heads of my wayward guests. Alberto towered over all of us somewhat proudly.

Their eyes looked at me unblinking, and they watched closely as I broke off a sprig of lemon basil, my fingers rolling the leaf then extending it outward, urging them to smell its fragrance. Apparently they took this as some sort of greeting, which I suppose it was, and mimicked my gesture. Deciding that my tour guide qualities were rapidly failing, I led them into the kitchen.

Their eyes scanned the room, gobbling in details like nutrients fueling their minds. I let them feed unhurriedly, with Alberto's obvious approval. Italians are big on gestures, so our inability to converse didn't seem insurmountable. The aroma of rosemary left over from last night's dinner hung in the air. I could see their curiosity mirrored in the glass jars lining the pantry shelves as they moved about the kitchen. I demonstrated what I could as they pointed to objects they wanted to know more about. A knife − for cutting; a faucet − to get water; water − for drinking, and so on. We were quite the harmonious little group unraveling mysteries − feeling, tasting, and smelling this community room.

They backed away from the light of the open refrigerator. This was clearly different from the cabinets which simply opened and shut, revealing hard surfaced flat or round things. Alberto madly scribbled away on his clipboard noting what these "guests" found amusing or interesting. When I saw the light distressed them, I groped inside the appliance blindly, searching for the heaviness of a round of Parmesan cheese. I brought it from behind my back and handed it to one of them with great expression in my face as if it were a huge surprise or treasure. Startled by its coolness, the alien dropped the cheese and we all watched as it rolled across the floor, halted by claw-like feet. I motioned for them to move aside as the *bruschetta* came out of the oven. I silenced my son's protest with a shush, and told him to hand me the cheese. Slicing off a hunk, I quickly grated it over the toasted bread and tomatoes. Shreds fell like raindrops and soon covered the red surface. All the while, almost a dozen eyes were watching.

Encouraging them with gestures to ape me once again, I leaned over the plate and inhaled with gusto. They did the same. I grasped one piece of the warm treat in my hand and hungrily took a bite. They did the same − although their "mouths" turned out to be what I'd thought up until then were their ears! See? I wanted to say to Alberto. You think you know so much. Look at them, these aliens of yours. They *love* the *bruschetta!*

I grinned with smug satisfaction at my big, smart, scientist son. Those nice aliens did the same.

It was all a mother could ask.

AFRAID OF OUR FOOD?

BY ELLEN NORDBERG

'd like the spinach salad," I say, quickly scanning the menu description for offensive ingredients. "Without the tomatoes and the croutons," I add.

The waiter fakes a smile. "Yah," he says, Boston accent leaking through the "h." The New England summer sun sprinkles light on our table through the oak trees above as I set my menu aside.

"Oh," I add. "And can you put the salad dressing on the side?"

My sister, a hotel school grad and ex-restaurant manager, shifts in her chair and re-opens her menu, shielding her expression. Our waiter turns his attention toward her.

"Instead of the chicken," I say. "Do you have tofu?"

"Tofu?" the waiter says, as if I have asked for frog brains or turtle poop to be sprinkled on my salad.

I guess not.

"Chicken is fine," I say. "And a cranberry juice with a splash of club soda and a lime."

The waiter chews on his lower lip and nods. "We have a cranberry spahklah drink that's already soda and cranberry mixed togetha," he offers.

"This sparkler drink, does it have sugar?" I say.

My sister leans toward me, and smiles apologetically at the waiter. She looks like she wants to shove me under the table, or perhaps bop me over the head with the whiffle bat she used on me periodically when we were in grammar school.

"Maybe I could try a sample," I say. "I'll bet it has sugar in it."

The waiter squints at me.

"I'm sorry," my sister tells him. "She can't help it; she's from L.A."

◇ ◇ ◇

"Oh my God!" the hostess of the holiday party says to a cluster of us standing by the food table in her dining room in West Hollywood. "All three of you look fabulous! So thin! What's the story?"

"Blood type diet," I say, picking up a broccoli floret. "I lost 10 pounds."

"Me too," the woman next to me in a tiny black velvet skirt adds. "I'm an O. No wheat. Low carbs."

"Yeah, it's great," the third woman says as the hostess nods intently. "I'm A. I feel so good after getting rid of red meat. I eat only soy products and rice pasta."

My friend Jo, in from Germany, snorts at us as she spreads Brie on a piece of sourdough bread.

"You know what Julia Child says," she asks.

We turn toward her, curious.

"You Americans!" she exhales heavily in a weird Euro accent, drawing in the deep gasping breaths so unique to Ms. Child. Jo swigs a big gulp of her white wine to enhance the imitation. "I've never met people," she breathes loudly, "so afraid of their food!"

◇ ◇ ◇

"No, no, no," my buddy Brad (the personal trainer) barks at our out-of-shape friend Bill. He slaps Bill's hand away from the breadbasket on the table in the café, then hands the full basket back to the busboy. "Bread is evil."

◇ ◇ ◇

I watch the *Raid Galoises* on the Outdoor Life Network. It's Europe's version of our Eco-Challenge, an event where handfuls of sicko athletes and ex-Marines slog through the jungle, rappel over waterfalls, mountain bike through rivers and run hundreds of miles through the desert – consecutively, and without sleep.

The cameras show the American team in camp: huddled over maps and compasses, doing calf stretches, eating specially formulated Power bar-type fuel, strategizing, gulping electrolyte-rich energy drinks.

Now we pan over the French camp: lounging lazily, chewing bloody steak, sipping red wine, and blowing smoke from European cigarettes.

Ha! I think. Those Americans will have the whole health/fitness/diet/workout thing engineered and wired. The French are smoking, for God's sake! I once clawed my way through a mini-triathlon in search of smaller thighs and am in awe of these hyper-fit competitors. I cozy down with some original Styrofoam flavor rice cakes to watch the Americans kick ass.

An hour later, 17 hours of footage having been condensed, I watch in amazement as the French cruise across the finish line in first place, looking fresh and rested. The Americans have wrenched an ankle. Someone is in tears.

◇ ◇ ◇

In the book *The Only Diet There Is*, author Sondra Ray suggests that our beliefs about food determine the effect it will have on our bodies. In other words, if we believe Twinkies will make us fat, they will. Or if we think chicken soup will help a cold, it does. I consider the winning French team, my friend Jo and Julia Child, and I wonder, am I afraid of my food?

I avoid alcohol, sugar, chocolate, and caffeine, not for fat purposes but because I fear them to be the culprit for 3 AM hysterical fights with what are now ex-boyfriends. I don't drink diet soda because I'm afraid it causes breast cancer. I avoid carbohydrates like bread and pasta to stay thin, and dairy products for reasons I cannot recall. I've been on the PMS diet, the Blood Type Diet, and Weight Watchers twice. On a hike in Bryce Canyon during my most anti-carb obsessed phase, I ended up in an emergency room in rural Utah with heatstroke and an IV in my arm due to eating only dry tuna wrapped in lettuce.

While claiming the more flattering excuse of health reasons for my behavior, between the mirror and myself I know vanity and body image are closer to the truth. But how much control is too much? Are there only two choices? Bread-obsessed fitness girl or undisciplined, out of breath, satisfied whale?

Is there a connection between our thoughts and what we eat? Maybe the custom of praying over food, setting the intention that whatever it is will be healing and healthy makes sense. Perhaps sugar in reasonable doses might not cause emotional meltdowns. Maybe bread with that tuna would give my muscles something to burn for a change. Maybe a handful of pretzels wouldn't cause an instant downward slide into brownies and vanilla ice cream hell. Maybe.

◇ ◇ ◇

My sister and I meet in Florida over a long weekend for our grandmother's ninetieth birthday. We sneak off one night together for dinner on an outdoor patio. The waiter approaches.

"Here we go," my sister says into her napkin, crossing one flip-flopped foot across the opposite thigh.

He hands each of us menus and asks for our drink orders.

I quickly scan the wine and beer list, sucking in a deep breath.

"I'll bet they don't have cranberry juice," my sister says, eyeing the waiter sympathetically.

"I'll have a Foster's beer!" I blurt out a little too loudly, like someone wearing headphones.

My sister looks at me.

"I'll have an Amstel Light," she tells the waiter, watching me sideways, foot jiggling the dangling flip-flop. Perhaps she is thinking I am not aware of the calories a Foster's contains, or that an alien has replaced me at our table.

I look over the menu like a bettor studying the sheets at the racetrack. The waiter walks away to get our drinks.

"And an order of fried mozzarella sticks!" I yell at his back.

My sister leans toward me in a sudden motion, mouth open, and pulls her chair closer into the table. Fried mozzarella sticks were our favorite in college after a hearty night of drinking. She smiles at me.

The waiter places our beers on the table.

"Cheers, mate," my sister says in a mock Australian accent.

"Cheers," I say.

The beer is fine, though not as cold as it could be. But the mozzarella sticks have the perfect crunchy fried breading, and strings of warm cheese wrap around my tongue as I bite down. I love cheese.

"Mmhmh," I say to my sister.

"Mmhmh," she says.

I make it through half the beer and two fried cheese sticks before my health conscience kicks in. My Capri pants feel tighter already and I'm afraid I'll be hung-over tomorrow. But it's a baby step toward minimizing my obsession with the perfect diet, the perfect body, the perfect health program.

In the ensuing months, I take more baby steps away from food fear. I eat Danish Havarti cheese at a party and popcorn at the movie theatre – but without butter. Maybe a beer and a few chicken wings at a bar with friends, or a few too many tortilla chips with a veggie burrito.

The new guy I'm seeing invites me to his family's home for Christmas dinner where they serve (horrors!) ham. But I eat it, grateful that we pray over the food beforehand, giving me a chance to set my intention: one slice of ham can be healing and healthy. My blood pressure will not immediately arc up through the vaulted ceiling.

I shy away from food conversations with girlfriends who go psychotic wearing size two jeans instead of size zero. I try to listen to my intuition, integrating what makes sense from the books and articles I've read rather than dogmatically applying new food theories without question. I'll never convince myself a Snickers bar isn't poison, but an occasional burger and fries tastes pretty satisfying, and seems to have no ill effect.

I'm still careful about eating too many bagels and chips and crackers and those fried air triangles at the Chinese restaurant, and feel better when I listen to my body and eat well. When I don't eat sugar, I do have fewer problems with PMS, but Pad Thai sure tastes like grass and dough without it.

It may be too soon for major pronouncements, but I think listening to myself and taking a more balanced approach toward eating gives me more energy for non-food related thoughts. My body feels stronger, and there have been no recent carbohydrate deficiency-induced trips to the ER. At the very least when dining with my sister, I'm sparing myself the whiffle bat.

SEAWEED AND SUSHI ON SATURDAY NIGHT

BY KIMBERLY G. O'LONE

No way could I move from the couch, but I knew I should phone Veronica about Saturday night. Although it was 7:00, I guessed she would still be at her office. I was right. "Is it still girls' night out Saturday?" I said.

"Of course; I e-mailed you about it last week."

"Oh...I haven't been checking lately. I called because I knew it was your turn to make the arrangements, and I was wondering if we could move it to brunch out here in the suburbs. I'm just so tired at night, now that I'm in my eighth month, and the drive into the city..."

Dead silence for a few long seconds. "Oh, Gale honey, I just can't. Saturday is my spa day. I've had this appointment at Georgette's for weeks. I absolutely need it. I start with a therapeutic massage, and a paraffin wax pedicure. Next, I get my eyebrows arched, an aroma therapy facial and a mini-makeover. I'm also getting a French manicure. Monsieur Gregory says it will look elegant. Oh, I almost forgot, I'm getting a skin pore reduction too. What do you think?"

Pore reduction, I thought. *At this stage I could use a breast reduction. And I can barely bend over to shave my legs.* What I said was, "Sounds great. So you're too busy for Saturday brunch. How's next week?"

"Sorry, I'm giving tours for the Architecture Foundation. And the week after I'm on a retreat with the Adult Discovery Center. I'm hoping to meet someone decent this time. If not this Saturday, I'm booked for two months."

I sighed. "I guess I could take a nap in the afternoon."

"If only I had that luxury," Veronica snapped back.

If only I still had the luxury of sleeping on my stomach, I thought.

"As I said in my E-mail," Veronica began, "Sally will pick you up at 6:30. I'll meet you two downtown at Nikko's. It's Japanese. *Chicago Magazine* says their sushi's the best."

"Sushi," I could not keep the doubt from my voice.

A pause resonated at the other end. "Last summer, you said it might be fun to try Japanese."

I wasn't pregnant then, I thought.

"I've set it all up, but I suppose I could cancel the reservations."

"No," said I softly, "It'll be fine." *And raw,* I thought.

"Good. Gotta go so I'm not late for Claude."

"Claude?"

"My personal trainer? The marathon?"

"Oh, of course," said I. "Bye." I heard the dial tone. *Marathon!* I thought, as I struggled to rise from the couch.

◇ ◇ ◇

Late Saturday afternoon I surfaced from deep sleep when my husband shook my arm. "What," I said, pulling the covers over my head.

"You told me to wake you for that dinner with those neurotic friends of yours tonight," Phil said, sitting down on the edge of the bed. "You OK?"

"Dinner," I said groggily. I used to look forward to these nights all month. But money would be tight with my upcoming maternity leave. "Of course. I'm getting up."

As I put on the same black dress I had worn to the Greek restaurant last month, I scowled, wishing I had something new. With only one month left, though, it didn't make sense to buy new clothes.

I strained as I got up into Sally's Custom Land Rover. I landed on the Corinthian leather seats with an ungraceful thud. Sally looked me up and down. "You're huge!" she said. "Are you sure you still have a whole month to go?"

"My doctor said so," I repeated my stock answer. I had been finding that everyone, from store clerks to distant cousins seemed compelled to tell me how big I was. Now I was getting it from my friends.

Sally talked – again – about how she'd been passed over for promotion as the director of the nursing home. I tried to listen, but by the time we had gone five miles toward our 22-mile venture to downtown Chicago, I was asleep. Sally woke me just before the valet took the Land Rover's keys.

Veronica was waiting at a table in the small bar at Nikko's, her full-length sable coat draped over a chair. After she hugged us both, she said, "I'm going to have to get an arm extension, you're so big." I forced a token smile. Veronica continued, "They're crowded tonight. I told the waiter we'd take a private room so we could get in right away. It cost $25 extra, but we're worth it."

I nodded weakly, wondering what the bill was going to be if it cost $25 just to sit down. As the waiter led us to our room, I noticed Veronica's aqua silk pantsuit, and again cursed my same old black maternity dress. Then I gasped when I saw the dining area. We would have to sit on mats on the floor! What about my aching back? If I got down there, how would I get up? With a Japanese crane?

Neither woman seemed to notice my discomfort as they removed their shoes. Sally squealed in delight at Veronica's red polished toes, exclaiming, "I was going to go red, but chickened out and went with 'Moonstruck Pink.'"

"It's 'Wanted Red or Alive,' Veronica said seriously, "I almost went with 'Red Rhapsody.' I had such a hard time deciding."

The smell of wet nail polish makes me sick now, I thought, as I quietly kicked off my shoes, trying not to call attention to my unpainted toes, and the fact that I could not bend down. Our tiny Japanese waiter noticed my plight. He tried not to totter as he helped me lower my pregnant bulk onto the mat.

Veronica and Sally had tall bottles of Sapporo beer, which I noticed were $12 each. I drank tonic water. Veronica, who'd ordered the main course based on the sushi recommendations of *Chicago Magazine,* said this was her last big meal before she began her new diet of kiwi and black coffee. "It's called the "Kwoffee," Veronica said enthusiastically. "Claude is worried it might not give me enough carbohydrates, but I told him that I just feel fat in a size seven."

I thought of the 60 pounds I had gained, adding to my discomfort as I shifted around on the mat. When my belly touched the table edge, the baby kicked, thrusting out a limb and shaking the table. Conversation ceased as waves rippled through their drinks.

"It's like an alien could burst out of there at any second!" said Veronica, staring at the baby belly.

I stared back icily. I was beginning to feel like I'd had enough of my friends' comments.

Sally broke the silence by launching into a discussion of movies, none of which I had seen. They were throwing around titles like *The End of an Affair* and *Anna and the King*. My mind began to wander. As my stomach growled I began to think about real food, American food, like a big juicy hamburger, or German food like my grandmother used to make; big plates of sausage.

I was brought back from my musings when the salad arrived, consisting of five kinds of seaweed mixed with slices of octopus. I picked around the tentacles. The main course included pearl sized bright orange fish eggs that popped when I tried to chew them, broiled seaweed with fried tofu, and monkfish liver. Gazing at the small table of tiny tidbits, I felt I was dining in a dollhouse.

As I took my Rolaids out, I was amazed I had managed to nibble at any of this food. My back ached miserably, but the meal was almost over. All that was left was the green-tea ice cream. Figures, I thought, in a restaurant where you can get raw fish served fifteen different ways, the only dessert would be green-tea ice cream? It looked like a ball of army green Play-Doh. Forget it.

When the bill came Veronica said, "With tip, it's $85 each."

I gasped.

"What's wrong," asked Sally.

"I didn't drink any beer."

Into the silence that followed Veronica said, "We've always just split the bill."

"But that was when I was drinking, too."

"She's right," said Sally. After staring at the bill a moment, she said, "It's $65 for Gale and $95 for each of us."

Veronica frowned, but pulled out extra bills.

An older Japanese man I took to be the headwaiter walked to our table. "Is there a problem? Are you feeling OK, ma'am?" He had a look of fear that I had begun to recognize. It was the 'oh my God, she's going to have the baby right here' look.

"We're fine." Veronica assured him, and gave him the cash. He returned with a very large Japanese man from the kitchen, a giant I thought could have been a Sumo wrestler if he'd worn fewer clothes. Together, the two men lifted me to my feet.

"We'll get you right home," Sally said as we moved out into the night air.

"No," said I, refreshed, "I'm hungry."

"Hungry," exclaimed the other two.

"Yeah. I wonder if that deli across the street is still open."

"There?" sniffed Veronica.

"I have to. I need a liver sausage sandwich." In answer to their confused looks I said, "Some people call it *braunschweiger.*"

Inside, a middle-aged waitress, smiled broadly. "You're carrying low," she said, motioning us to a table and handing me the menus. "Looks like a boy to me."

I smiled back, feeling comfortable for the first time in hours. "We won't know until it comes out." I said. "I like surprises."

"The best way," agreed the waitress as she wiped the intended table clean. "My daughter just had her first. A girl. She insisted on knowing. She wanted the ultrasound, the amniocentesis, the works."

"Really," I said, "I skipped the amnio. The idea of putting a needle in my belly, well, I just did *not* want to do it. And there *is* some risk to the baby."

"*Just* what I told her, but thank God, she had a healthy girl."

I noticed that the others had fallen into their own conversation. Both ordered coffee without ever opening their menus, then resumed debating which singles party they should go to on Valentine's Day. I didn't care about joining in anymore. By Valentine's Day, if all went well, I would be celebrating with my husband and our new baby. *Our new baby,* I thought, still absorbing the dream come true.

When the waitress brought the order, she paused, coffeepot in hand. "So have you had an easy time of it, honey?"

"Hardly," I began, sitting back and resting my hands on my watermelon-sized abdomen. "But tell me, did the hospital ask your daughter to donate her placenta?"

Veronica momentarily stopped sipping her coffee.

"As a matter a fact, yes."

"To help cancer patients," I said, my mouth full. "It makes sense. It's full of special nutrients. I learned on the Web that some midwives cut and dry their clients' placentas like beef jerky. Then they grind the meat into a powder and put it into capsules for the mothers. They say it stimulates milk production when you eat your own placenta."

Veronica choked. *Who cares,* I thought, eating lustily and wiping ketchup from my chin. I was no longer on their wavelength, that was clear. The only thing I cared about that moment was that thick sandwich, the best liver sausage sandwich I had ever, ever eaten.

TOO PO' T' TOTE IT

BY LEANA PAGE

ate so much I feel too po' t' tote it," said Mavis as she yanked on the elastic waistband of her jogging pants and stretched it into a new position.

"Say what?" said Lillie. "Girlfriend, you keep forgetting I was born up North."

"The folks from the old country used to say that old stuff after they'd eaten everything in sight: too po' t' tote it," said Mavis.

For 30 years they'd carried on like this, so this particular day after Thanksgiving was no different. Except for maybe more Tupperware piled up than usual.

"Old country? You mean like Mississippi?

"Yeah, did you think I was talking Europe?"

"Say it again." Lillie said. "You're talking too fast."

"Too po' t' tote it," teased Mavis as she spoke the words with a slight degree of speed.

"Would you please translate for me? I was born right over there at Michael Reese Hospital," said Lillie.

"Well, your mama was raised down South."

"No fair talking about my mama." A cloud briefly crossed her face.

"Your problem's not your mama, it's that you're listening too slow. Listen faster and keep up: too po' t' tote it."

Lillie strained to understand.

"Girl, it's when you eat so much you're overloaded, you know, bloated, heavy. Too poor to tote it." She enunciated each word with exaggeration. "Too weak to carry all that heavy soul food," said Mavis. "You know, especially at times like Christmas, weddings." She paused. "And funerals, where all the people who pitched in, helping some soul on his way finally got to sit down all together and eat a meal, remembering him." Suddenly the hollows in her gaunt face deepened. "How is your mama? Seriously."

Lillie shrugged. "Good days, bad days."

Mavis bit her lower lip, knowing so well what that meant as she recalled her own recovery from breast cancer less than a year before. It was just another flashback of the many weeks filled with nausea, weakness and a dangerous lightheadedness throughout the radiation and chemo treatments. Her usual dark cocoa colored skin had taken on an unnatural smutty hue during that time. Her salvation had been her good friend Lillie waiting in the doctor's office to drive her home after each treatment. If it hadn't been for her, she'd have curled up into a little ball in bed and simply wasted away.

"Kinda like Cleo," Lillie said.

No, Mavis thought – *not Cleo* – *not now. How long can I –*

As if reading her mind Lillie interrupted her thoughts with "How're you making out with your doctors?"

She met Lillie's gaze, then looked down at her plate. "Right now..." She paused, gathering her resources. "Sure, it was benign last week, but it wasn't last year, and who knows about next year, if..." Her sigh resounded from the high-ceilinged room. "I see my fate in her."

"She wants to see you," Lillie said softly as she reached to take Mavis' hand. She turned her grasp into loving caresses as she lowered her head, shaking it slowly from side to side. "I know how hard this is for you, but maybe I can make it a little easier for her – or her family. You do what you feel comfortable doing." Lillie paused as she searched for the right words. "Sometimes you just have to pack up your troubles and move them to the side. I know you're still trying to find your way back. So – whatever's best for you."

"You know, I'm trying. But it's like every day I start out at ground zero. I still have to force myself to think positive. That's what she has to do – think positive." Mavis caught herself, blinked, and stopped. "But she won't be – no – she won't." She cleared her throat. "She won't be getting better. Life is just running out on her."

"You need more dressing?" Lillie rose abruptly and reached for the nearest Tupperware. It was so good to see Mavis' appetite had returned. Still, she remained rail thin with a slight paunch below the waist. Just last year she had been plump and voluptuous.

Mavis exhaled, relieved at the diversion. "I really shouldn't; but Girlfriend, you really put your foot off in this dressing. It tastes just like the stuffing my mother made – almost a meal by itself," she said as she forked more food into her mouth. With every lift of her head she swung her thick cornrow braids out of the way, and with closed eyes she praised the food with an "Oomph Oomph" deep down in her throat so as not to interrupt the flow of food.

"I love good dressing too," said Lillie as she stifled the urge to confess the tears that had salted it Wednesday night. Tears that came from knowing it was probably the last holiday for Cleo, her best friend from the first time they'd seen each other at the Frances E. Willard Elementary School's First Grade. They'd met Mavis in third grade, becoming a trio. She pivoted sharply on one foot and turned to her friend, a wicked grin on her face. "And please, Girl, do not – do not – call my dressing stuffing. Stuffing is that junk they push up into the turkey's behind hoping it'll make the bird taste like something."

"Every year I ask you what you put in it."

"You know I don't have a real, written recipe. It's always different. I just work with it until I get it to taste a certain way. I didn't learn to make it with a measuring cup. My old folks cooked with a pinch of this and smattering of that. That's how I learned, you know, by touch and taste. I mean it depends on certain main ingredients. Heavy on the corn bread, and toasted day-old bread to fill in the blank spots. I always get extra chicken livers and gizzards and boil them in finely diced onion, celery and green pepper. You see, it's the broth that you use to bind it with."

"And here I thought it was the eggs."

Lillie laughed.

"Yeah, and these biscuits almost melt in your mouth," Mavis said. "I could almost eat six of these bad boys."

"Looks like you already ate eight or nine of them. And do not call my rolls biscuits," chided Lillie.

"I'll call them anything you want me to if you just tell me how you made them."

"Actually, Mama made the rolls," confessed Lillie.

Mavis' eyebrows raised questioningly.

"Wednesday was one of her better days, so she baked them. But still, Alzheimer's ... well, I've learned to simply revel in her good days. Now, today though, she's shut up in her room, nodding off every five minutes when she's not thinking she's back in Mississippi."

"Still, you've had her all these years," said Mavis, trying to recall being someone's daughter. She had been motherless now for nearly 20 years. "You can cook and bake with her, and then eat it..."

"Food's always best when you share it. You need someone to play off of. There's no need to go 'Mmmm' if there's no one there to hear it," said Lillie, looking around the room that had become so familiar to her over the years. "Like anything in life, it should be shared."

"Bad news just like the good?" She cut herself a generous slice of pumpkin spice cake.

"Whatever life brings." Lillie walked across the room and opened a cabinet. As she reached up to the highest shelf of the cabinet, she stretched her cinnamon colored body, slim despite all her time spent fixing food. It had only been in the last few years that she had moved reluctantly from a single digit size to an overflowing size ten. She'd absolutely forbidden herself to get any bigger. From the top shelf she pulled down another throw away deli container, easy with her 5' 10" frame.

Mavis looked down at her own body, thin and wasted from bouts of chemo and radiation. "I think about that biopsy last week," she said as felt the hot needle of fear shoot through her, sharp as a biopsy needle. With a puzzled look on her face she said, "I got a pass this time. It was benign. I still haven't figured out why I'm here."

"To eat up all my food," teased Lillie as a Cheshire grin spread across her bony face. She, too, was relieved.

"I have a lot of cancer time to make up for. Who knows how much time I have left, so you know I'm goin' for it," said Mavis as she looked around the kitchen that looked much the same as the first day she'd come home with Lillie all those years ago.

Lillie's sigh came from deep within as she gazed out the window. "Yeah. Cleo's just about quit eating. Her family's nearly at wits end with worry and exhaustion. They've insisted upon keeping her home where she wants to be. At the rate her cancer's been spreading since it got into her lymph nodes, well..." she took a long breath. "With her mom having congestive heart failure these five years – "

Mavis finished her sentence. "And now it looks like Cleo will go before her. Go figure. What about her brothers?"

"They just don't get it. I think more than anything they'll get in the way from here on out. Some men have such a hard time understanding these things. They've barely gotten a grasp on living."

"No, I think they understand. They just have a hard time expressing what they really feel. Why are they so different?"

"My mother once told me," Lillie said as she shoveled dressing into a large Tupperware and firmly sealed it, "that it's because mothers raise their daughters and love their sons."

"Ain't that the truth," said Mavis with a chuckle followed by a thoughtful frown. "We learn to accept things easier and move along with the flow." She paused. "How do you die? How does anybody die?" Hesitantly she reached across the table and placed her hand on Lillie's arm, her other hand still holding a forkful of cake.

Lillie turned to her friend. "One day at a time, one triumph at a time, one failure at a time. Dying starts the day you're born – or maybe the day you decide to just let go."

"I think letting go is the worst – no, the hardest, thing we will ever do."

Lillie nodded. "Seems so for Cleo – she's still talking about going to Bobby's graduation, and we're all amazed she's made it through Thanksgiving."

"And you two - best of friends since first grade."

"And you too, Girlfriend. You know I love you both."

Mavis smiled her appreciation.

"She was telling me the other day how she could feel her body just shutting down on her. Her mind is still in fast mode, while her body has stopped doing what she wants it to," said Lillie, clearing away some of the dishes.

"I'm so glad she had a second chance at love with Henry. Now that's a good man."

"Yeah, he's really hanging in there and I know it has to be hard for him," Lillie said quietly.

"So now what – we just wait?" said Mavis.

"I figure I can alternate evenings going in to visit and just plain pick up the slack. It might make her time a little more bearable."

"How's her spirits?"

"Good. In fact, she laughed when I said if she gets to heaven before me she's got to scout everything out. That'll make my transition easier."

"I'm not so sure about where I'll be going..." Mavis frowned.

"Yeah, but for the moment you know where you are. Live. Laugh. Eat. Hey – you want some more of this stuff before I put it away?"

Mavis' face brightened. "Well, you could fix me a plate to take with me."

"Why don't you do that yourself? You can use my throw away Tupperware. Over in that corner are all those containers from the deli I've been saving. That way you won't have to return them to me. I learned a long time ago not to let folks take my good stuff out of here," said Lillie with the voice of a wise old woman.

"Girl, you got more 'good stuff' than you know what to do with," said Mavis as she looked around the kitchen big enough to cater food for the whole neighborhood. "You've been such a good friend to Cleo. A lot more than me. But I will – " she broke off her words in mid-sentence. "I will go to see her – tomorrow. Will you be there, too?"

"Listen, you've had you hands full with your own illness," she said, her eyes warm with understanding. "Would you believe, Cleo talked about maybe going Christmas shopping downtown tomorrow? And who's to say she won't? Maybe it's her way of getting ready –"

"To let go?"

"Yeah, to let go. Her family's wiped out. If she goes shopping anywhere, it'll be because you and I take her," Lillie said.

"I remember my mama telling me – right toward the end, you know – that she'd wanted to go shopping over the weekend, and that her friends from church took her, right after the service. She told me on a Monday, and she died the next day."

"The old folks – they knew how to do for each other."

"Still do. Not only in the old country, but here, too. And with food for every occasion. You, know after a funeral they have one of those things, you know, a repast. They make a big feast for the family to enjoy after they've been to the cemetery. It makes it easier for them to get back to the world around them, make jokes and remember the deceased. But you never leave all by yourself." She faltered. "I mean you're alone – but not by yourself, and with letting go – well, we just get too po' t' tote it all by ourselves, and we need someone in our corner, a friend to lean on. We just need people in our lives."

"You want to go tomorrow?"

"Where, Girlfriend? Shopping?"

"Yeah, let's take Cleo shopping. Even if we only get her to one store and she just buys a single thing, it'll be better then nothing. And if she's up to it, we'll do more."

"I'll bet she buys out the store," said Mavis as she fought to lighten the conversation.

"And she'll need someone to help her tote it."

She grinned. "City Girl, you say 'tote' like you've been saying it all your life."

BEAN FIEND

BY CAROLYN PAPROCKI

Screaming for beans,
My morning caffeine,
Got to get those beans.

Beans pouring out like a slot machine;
Mocha java jackpot –
Choose your flavor,
The one to savor,
Got to get those beans.

One cup won't do;
Got to have two,
Or I get mean,
'Cause I'm hooked on the bean,
Hooked on the bean.

My hands are shaking,
My head's a-twirl,
This caffeine's got me in a whirl;
My knees are knocking,
My nerves are bare,
This stuff is bad,
You think I care?

Breakfast's over, but I can't wait,
For that good old time
Called the coffee break,
'Cause I got a habit I just can't shake;

I'm a bean fiend,
A bean fiend.

VIRGINIA'S BIRTHDAY DINNER

BY DORIS J. POPOVICH

 veryone always thought Virginia and Isabel were twins. Understandably so. Their physical resemblance was striking, mirrored images, really – and their likeness didn't stop there. They were both shy and a little stubborn, preferring Mama's corn bread to conversation. The only things they loved more than Grandma's apple pie were each other.

On May 2nd, 1910, Virginia's 9th birthday, which coincidentally fell on exactly the same day as Isabel's 8th birthday, Isabel and Virginia decided to be twins, agreeing it would be easier than correcting everyone about it for the rest of their lives. The following year, Isabel and Virginia celebrated their 9th birthday, Virginia for the second time. Friends and family never protested, though as the years passed, some thought it odd.

◇ ◇ ◇

Isabel knew the truth about herself, and she knew right from wrong, but the truth had not set her free. Instead it divided her inner landscape like a crack divides a mirror, like pain divides a day.

The kitchen was quiet except for the imminent moan of simmering turnip greens, and a distant clock ticking. She steadied herself against the old Roper stove, unearthed the salt pork, then forced a hot splash when she dropped it back in again, remembering how Virginia loved her greens bitter salty.

Dumplin's, fried gizzards, greens and craklin' bread, Virginia's hundredth birthday dinner. Just like they'd talked about, last time they'd talked. Just like she'd promised.

Her ruminations about God's will were interrupted by a knock at the door. Paramedics too young to understand wheeled Virginia to the bedroom. Papers were signed and Sunday's return trip to the Methodist Home arranged.

Isabel returned to the kitchen and prepared a plate for each of them. En route to the bedroom she stopped by the oven and blew out both pilot lights, leaving the oven and four burners turned on high.

"Happy Birthday, Sis." She spoke for both of them. Then she began feeding Virginia dinner.

DIGGING OUT ON POETRY
(AT THE 7TH ANNUAL WOODLAND MARATHON)

BY NANCY F. RAFAL

A feast planned for early afternoon to far into the night,
invited poets' prepared concoctions set before a salivating audience,
people come and go, go and come, a few stay and stay.

Ten readers an hour, then a ten minute break,
a procession of word platters to please all tastes,
light tangy morsels sprinkled throughout.

Spicy works to stir your senses,
cozy comforts recalling universal yesterdays,
stinging bitter bites warning of daze to come.

White wine words, merlot, the hard stuff,
a few boilermakers, local suds on tap,
soft drink sips, a low-cal here and there.

A taste of home, exotic herbs, ripe fruit,
tough talk to chew and chew,
a taste of blood, a rose, a rose, a rose.

Just desserts, some sweet, some savory,
trifle, a pudding plum,
bitter chocolate, Jell-O, too.

And when the feast is finished, and all
have licked the platters clean, I can only say,
"Please pass the poetry; there's always
room for more."

TURKEY

BY K.S. ROSENTHAL, M.D.

urkeys are funny looking. As adults, that is — cuz as poults they look a lot like chicks and they peep like chicks when they're lonely. This was our first turkey. We bought him with Thanksgiving in mind, and one turkey seemed right enough for a family of three. Besides, I had heard turkeys were aggressive and nasty as adults, stupid, foul creatures who bit at one's ankles when a broom wasn't handy. But raising a sole turkey made for a lonely turkey, and Grandma carried him about in her bra, between her breasts, keeping him warm and happy. Grandma had Alzheimer's and often forgot he was there — "My GOD! Kimmy! Who put this little bastard in my bra!" Then she'd grow soft a minute later. "Ach, never mind. Leave the poor thing where he is." We had chicks, too. You're not supposed to raise chicks and poults together — turkeys catch chicken diseases and die very quickly — but this lonely turkey cried all night and every night, and something had to be done.

At first we kept him indoors at night. He slept with Grandma, who started to remember some things about turkeys, and things went well until he grew cumbersome and gangly and too big to fit between her breasts. My husband put his foot down. "I don't care if it kills him. He needs to stay outside with the other chickens."

So Turkey became a chicken. He roosted with them, took sand baths like them, and raided the neighbor's vegetables. Grandma chuckled when she saw him. "He'll taste good, that turkey," she said. Often Turkey stood outside the window, turning his head left and right, watching us and trying to sneak inside when a door was accidentally left open. Sometimes he lost the other chickens and whooped sadly until I helped him find them. Turkey became part of the family. How could anything that had slept with Grandma and sat between her breasts be considered a meal? He was left alone and gained weight accordingly. At about 40 pounds he developed a right-sided hip dysplasia. There he was, my turkey, limping about and standing on his left leg like a flamingo. Soon he couldn't walk. By early November he stayed in the chicken pen all the time. I carried him out in the mornings to sit in the sun.

"Don't worry," my grandma said. "All turkeys get depressed about this time of year. He'll get over it." We fed him bits of bread and stroked his beak and neck to help him sleep. I carried him about on the wheelbarrow and he spent the nights in Grandma's room. They both sat under the tree during the day: she in her wheelchair, and he on his wheelbarrow. "Good meal, that turkey," insisted Grandma. Turkey never did get better. "Turkeys aren't meant to weigh 40 pounds," said my neighbor. He was thinking of his vegetables, maybe. "Their little legs can't take it. Cruel to let him go on that way." We watched and waited. Watched and waited. Turkey limped about on occasion, but got no better. He cried most of the time. I gave him a couple of shots of Grandma's best coffee brandy, topped that off with a bit of tequila, and gave him to my neighbor.

Birds don't tolerate alcohol well. Turkey had liked the taste of coffee brandy and guzzled it up over a slice of bread, but he grew weary and top-heavy and soon fell dead asleep. I suppose intoxication was a nice way to go. Anyway the neighbor was happy and carried him off in a large box. They invited us to dinner and we ate him over a barbecue. Grandma forgot Turkey quickly. But I didn't. How could I forget anything that had slept with Grandma and sat between her breasts? Granted, he didn't taste too good. "Too dry, this turkey," agreed Grandma, and she refused to eat any more of him.

A Taste for It

by Deborah Dashow Ruth

No one ever taught me to eat
a poem slowly, to take small bites
and make it last, so I just
cram the whole damn thing
in my mouth, too impatient
to let the flavors linger
or allow my taste buds to savor
the tang. I gulp lines, choke
on enjambment, and bite down
so hard on imagery, I get
similes stuck between my teeth.
Sometimes I even swallow a poem
without chewing it, and wonder
why my tongue goes numb.

FOOD THAT RIDES OFF INTO THE SUNSET

BY LYNN VEACH SADLER

I've been warned by very wise people,
both literati and denizens of Grub Street,
never to write poems about food.
(At least the latter, I find quite remarkable.)
But, then, I've never taken a warning wisely, assuredly,
and have always been right full of beans.

So if I were to slip and write (right?) such a poem—
I'd indulge in MY FANTASY MENU, eat it right (write?)
back to a favorite time, place, and table.

Saloon Hour? *Gabby Hayes Roasted Peanuts,*
Cisco Kid Salsa and Pancho Chips
wet down with *Red Disturbance.*
"Happy Trails" Salad (Greens, Red Onion, Avocado,
Orange Segments, and "Ranch" Dressing).
Lone Ranger Mesquite-Flavored Steamship Round.
Mexican Spitfire Chicken Enchiladas.
Lash La Rue Sweet Potatoes (with "Whipped" Butter,
Cinnamon, Brown Sugar, and Secret Lillie Gilder).

Judge Roy Bean Pintos with Lillie Langtry Condiments
(Green Onions, Tomatoes, Green Pepper, Cilantro).
Cochise Corn Bread.
Smiley Burnette Blueberry Cobbler.
Eschewing greenhorns, I'd swap Steamship Round for
cattaloe, Texas longhorn, Sonora red, or zorrilla.
Entertainment? LILLIE LANGTRY,
THE FAMOUS OPERA SINGER
ADORED BY THE FAMOUS HANGING JUDGE,
JUDGE ROY BEAN.
Flowers? Plain "Jersey Lilies," no fancy fluff-duff.
Conversation? We'd chew on "op'ra house"
as the corral fence's top rail,
where cowboys more or less
talked over the few things they talked over.
Benediction? *Adios, Amigos, until we eat again.*

WHO AM I?

BY TRINIDAD SÁNCHEZ, JR.

Am I
the collection of pinto beans,
the pile of warm *tortillas*
the *chile relleno*, the *tostada* chip
dipped in your *salsa picante.*
The *flautas* you eat with your *dedos,*
the chocolate *con canela,*
the *nopales*, the *salchichas*
you so richly savor?

Am I
the oregano, the cilantro, *la cebolla*
of your *salsa bien picosa,*
the *jalapeño* peppers
the *pimienta* in your *gazpacho?*
Let's be honest - it's true . . .
I did say: *Me gustan las gorditas!*
I also said: I loved your *chilaquiles!*

Am I
the super nacho of your life
or will I only be the rice and beans
forever?

Yo sé bien, you don't like to joke around
at times you think of me as a *taco de carbon!*
Where's the beef?
You would do well to teach
your Mexican sandwich *Español*
pa'que no pierda su identidad
and become Hispanic, better yet . . .
Let him be CHICANO!

Sí, sí, I want to be
the *pan de huevo* you bite into,
the *calabaza* of your *empañada,*
the papa of your *papa con huevos,*
the sugar in your *atole!*

Ay Mamacita!
The two of us are made for each other
like *arroz con leche*
the *tamal* wrapped in the *hoja*
the extra *queso* on your *enchilada*
and all you can say is:

What's for dessert?

TONGUE IN JOWL

BY WHITNEY SCOTT

 everal years ago at the Lincoln Park's Farm in the Zoo, I saw eight piglets suckling at their mom, a huge motionless sow. She lay on her side with eyes closed in either blissful relaxation or the complete exhaustion of a mother who could no longer bear the constant demands of so many babies. Each tiny pig, on the other hand, poked and pushed, jockeying for position and sucking intently, some making little grunting sounds.

"Aren't they adorable," I said.

You smiled appreciatively. "Dinner – baby back ribs."

Justifiably alarmed, all eight stopped nursing and looked up, their eyes wide with fear.

"It's okay," I reassured them. "She doesn't mean it."

You leaned your 5' 8" frame over the guardrail. "YUM!" you said. Even Mama Sow opened her one visible eye at that, and the little pigs crowded closer to her, as though trying to burrow their way into her ample body for safety. She groaned in protest.

"Really, she's kidding – she is." A zookeeper over by the pygmy goats looked over, his eyes narrowed in suspicion. Apparently, he'd mistaken me for you, the insensitive carnivore standing to my right.

"No. I'm not," you insisted. "Not kidding at all. Mini pork roasts – Mmm. Mmmmm." You licked your lips.

One baby squealed in terror, and another, and another, then five tiny pink mouths howled in unison.

I sighed, shook my head, and turned to you. "Can't take you anywhere," I said.

PASS THE PASTA, PLEASE:
FROM GENERATION TO GENERATION

BY ROSEMARY SERLUCA

hen I'm gone, who's gonna get up and cook, eh?" my grandmother Rosina would ask in her Italian-accented English. "Nobody, that's who! You all gonna starve to death."

Every Sunday morning at 6:30, my grandmother, a short, chunky woman with a robust face, and coal-black hair worn in a tight bun, would sneak into her sanctuary – a small kitchen replete with avocado-green appliances, Formica countertops, and a buckling, beige, linoleum floor. In here, from such simple offerings as flour, eggs, and water, Nonna (as she insisted on being called) would create a venerable blessing – homemade pasta. I, at the age of five, would often join her, watching in wonderment, listening with ardor, learning the strength of family, and the gift of love.

"In *Italia*, during the war," she'd recount, "all I could make for my family was pasta. It's all we had."

She believed that by filling the bellies of her family members with something as hearty as her homemade pasta, she was providing a solid foundation from which to draw strength and courage.

Clasping her hands and emphatically shaking them, she'd say, "Back then, life was very hard, but we have each other. My pasta keep everybody strong, and everybody happy. And you know something? We survive."

Nonna began her revered ritual by putting on her special heirloom – a frayed, pink and yellow apron that had almost completely faded to white, save for the stains etched long ago from her mother's cooking. My Aunt Francesca tried to replace it once by giving her a set of crisp new aprons at Christmas.

"Are you crazy?" Nonna said, opening the box. "What are you tryin' to do, eh? Bring bad luck to my cooking with these things?

Take 'em back." Back they went, and the tattered relic lived on, Nonna refusing to cook without it.

Next, she would tune her tinny transistor radio to a program that featured the mellifluous voice of Mario Lanza. With the great lyric tenor singing "Be My Love," Nonna poured flour atop an oversized wooden cutting board and rhythmically shaped it into a ring. Into the empty center went the eggs and water.

With her strong, soft hands, Nonna mashed everything together, transforming the mixture into dough. Huffing and puffing, she'd knead it with her knuckles and palms, shaping it into a ball. I was given the fun job of raising the ball high over my head and slamming it on to the table, where it landed with a listless thud.

"Not like that, Bella," Nonna coached. "Like this."

She showed me the "correct" method, which was to knead the dough, lift it into the air and shout, "*Madonna buona,*" as it thumped down onto the table. Knead, lift, slam, and bless. Knead, lift, slam, and bless. It became our mantra. We repeated it six times in a row, blessing louder and louder at each slam.

"If they can't hear you," she'd say, looking up at the ceiling, "they can't help you. Bless with a big strong voice, and for sure you make a perfect pasta."

After a while, my role as assistant began to lose appeal. It was forcing me to miss my favorite TV show, "Wonderama" — a two and half hour children's program comprised of spelling bees, sing-a-longs, kids dancing on giant blocks, furry snakes popping out of tin cans, and a large treasure chest filled with toys and prizes. Host Bob McCallister was surrounded by a bevy of studio kids who would wave their arms in and out, high above their heads like air traffic controllers, vying for the camera's attention. My cherished dream was to be seen on national television, my arms flailing to and fro alongside my new TV pals.

As I sat just inches from the set, waving my right hand and blowing kisses with my left to the imaginary camera that had singled *me* out, I experienced an obtrusive broadcast interruption — Nonna marched right in front of the television set and blocked my view.

"It's two weeks you no help me, *Signorina,*" she reported. "If you no learn how to make pasta the right way, how you gonna live, eh?"

With my arms staying in complete sync with Bob and the gang, I flatly replied, "No big deal, I'll eat peanut butter and jelly sandwiches."

She grabbed her rosy cheeks with the palms of her beefy hands and shook her head in disbelief.

"*Mamma mia!* Peanut butter and the jelly? Together?" she shouted. "That's terrible!"

She never could bear to watch me delight in that combination, which to her, was "bad, bad American fake food."

Nonna squinted her eyes and pointed her index finger; she seemingly peered into my future and made an eerie prediction: "When you are a big girl, you gonna have to make pasta. If you no learn now, you gonna have big trouble later."

"Grandma! Come on, I can't see the TV!" I whined.

In a huff, she moved aside, bent down, and whispered slowly into my ear, "I see big trouble, *Signorina*. Big Trouble."

Nonna always claimed that she could "see" things, experience visions in her mind's eye that mere mortals could not. Once, when I couldn't find my Betsy Wetsy doll, Nonna closed her eyes and said she saw a vision of the doll stuck under the sofa bed. Sure enough Betsy was jammed in there, eyes wide open, waiting to be rescued. With my habit of leaving toys strewn about for Nonna to trip over, it never occurred to me that she might have stuffed poor Betsy there to teach me a lesson.

Giving absolute credence to her psychic ability, I took her prescient warning of a future riddled with "*Big Trouble*" to heart, and realized it would be in my best interest to pay more attention. I waved good-bye to Bob and the kids and quickly resumed my assistant's role in the kitchen.

By way of reward, I was allowed to flatten the dough with a large rolling pin. Nonna placed her protective hands over mine, and together we flattened the dough ball into what looked like the thinnest pizza I'd ever seen. We then set it on a tablecloth to dry for about 10 minutes.

Next, she'd roll it like a giant cigarette. With a long sharp knife, she'd slice horizontally across, creating the pasta of choice by cutting it thick or thin. Strips of spaghetti (thin), linguini (thicker), or fettuccine (thickest) would magically unravel. The long pieces of pasta fringe were draped over a wooden pole balanced between two kitchen chairs for 15 minutes. When the strips felt dry, they were ready for the big boil.

As the pasta swirled in a large aluminum pot, the "gravy" – as Nonna called her tomato sauce – bubbled alongside, releasing a redolent scent of herbs and spices. The aroma traveled up the stairs, through the hallway, and into the vestibule to greet my relatives, who arrived every Sunday at 1:00 PM to feast at Nonna's banquet. Following the seductive smell of garlic into the kitchen, they would consume an entire loaf of soft, mushy bread by dipping small chunks into the gurgling gravy. This pre-dinner plunging of bread would naturally upset Nonna.

She grimaced. "How you gonna enjoy my pasta if you eat so much bread, eh? You *need* my pasta to live. In *Italia*, everybody sit and *wait* for pasta."

My Uncle Luigi, a Sunday regular, was about to pop a delicious, gravy-soaked piece of bread into his mouth when she shouted, "Luigi! What are you doing, eh? Stop that! No more bread!"

Like a private being reprimanded by his general, Uncle Luigi immediately put the bread down, but when Nonna turned her back to him, he just couldn't resist the forbidden treat. He winked at me and ate it anyway.

Nonna's concern would prove completely unfounded, for there was never a problem with being too full to eat her savory pasta. We inhaled every last fringy piece, and wiped the gravy lingering in our bowls with even *more* bread. Throughout the convivial clamor of these Sunday dinners, Nonna sat at the very end of the table, full of pride and satisfaction, watching, as her family fed upon the most gracious expression of her love.

Many years have passed since my pasta-making classes with Nonna. The Sunday ritual of eating the homemade meal together as a family is now reserved for holidays only. But that does not stop my grandmother. At the age of 82, she still occasionally rises early on Sunday morning, puts on her apron – a new one finally, sent especially from her sister in Italy – and makes her offering. Except none of us has time to sit and eat together. We pack, wrap, stack, and take the food home.

On a recent visit, I asked Nonna how she felt about that.

"Not so good," she replied despondently. "Nobody come to eat my pasta on Sunday no more. Everybody busy. Gotta do this. Gotta do that. A long time ago, nobody busy. We sit and eat together. Everybody happy. Everybody strong."

She gazed her ebony eyes thoughtfully into mine. "Maybe nobody need me to make the pasta?" she said. "Maybe, I stop, eh?"

I wrapped my arms around her, assuring we needed her to keep this tradition alive, now more than ever.

"We need to eat your pasta, Nonna, just as much you need to make it."

She gently took my hand into hers. "Remember when you were a little girl? You love my kitchen."

"Of course I remember," I said, "slamming and blessing the dough, how could I forget? But my favorite is when you predicted I would have big trouble in my life if I didn't learn how to make pasta."

"Good," she said chuckling, "I'm glad you remember, because today, I'm too tired to cook. Roll up your sleeve *Signorina*, and you show *me* what I teach *you*, eh? And here, put this on. It's not my mother's, but it will bring you good luck."

Tying the propitious apron around my waist, I discovered my palms were sweaty, the pupil being carefully watched by the master during a sacred rite of passage.

"I don't know," I said sheepishly, "it's been a long time."

"Ah!" she shouted, clapping her hands, "it's just like I say. Big..."

"...Trouble," I said, cutting her off.

Now I'm not someone who can easily resist a challenge, especially one that, according to Nonna, was so powerful it could control my destiny. Wiping my clammy hands, I took a deep breath, and, to my surprise, began maneuvering those eggs and flour like an old pro. I even managed to hum a few bars of my grandmother's favorite tune. Mr. Lanza would be proud.

"*Brava*," my grandmother said, as I proceeded to knead, lift, slam and bless. "Just bless a little bit louder, and it looks like you no gonna have big trouble after all."

NONNA'S TRADITIONAL HOMEMADE PASTA
SERVES 4

5 CUPS ALL-PURPOSE FLOUR
4 LARGE EGGS
1/2 CUP WATER

- POUR THE FLOUR ONTO A CUTTING OR PASTRY BOARD IN A CIRCULAR SHAPE, MAKING A HOLE IN THE MIDDLE. IT SHOULD LOOK LIKE A GIANT BAGEL.
- BREAK THE EGGS INTO THE EMPTY CENTER, AND BEAT THEM WITH AN EGG WHISK.
- MIX THE FLOUR WITH THE EGGS AND SHAPE THE MIXTURE INTO A BALL.
- KNEAD THE DOUGH FOR ABOUT 5 MINUTES UNTIL IT'S SMOOTH.
- SPRINKLE SOME ADDITIONAL FLOUR ONTO THE BOARD, AND PLACE THE BALL OF DOUGH ONTO IT.
- WITH A ROLLING PIN, FLATTEN THE DOUGH UNTIL IT BECOMES AS THIN AS A PIZZA. (AS YOU ROLL, MOVE YOUR HANDS OUT FROM THE CENTER.)
- DRY FLATTENED DOUGH ON A CLEAN TABLE CLOTH OR TOWEL FOR ABOUT 10 MINUTES.

◇

- WITH YOUR HANDS, ROLL THE DOUGH AS IF ROLLING A CIGARETTE.
- WITH A LONG SHARP KNIFE, SLICE SHAPES AS IF CUTTING A STALK OF CELERY. THE TIGHTER YOU SLICE, THE THINNER THE PIECES. (IE. FOR SPAGHETTI SLICE VERY CLOSE TOGETHER, FOR LINGUINI SLICE FARTHER APART, FOR FETTUCCINE SLICE EVEN FARTHER.) FOR THOSE OF YOU THAT ARE NOT MANUALLY INCLINED, A PASTA MACHINE WILL DO JUST FINE.
- HANG THE PASTA ON A PASTA RACK TO DRY FOR ABOUT 15 MINUTES. (IF A PASTA RACK IS NOT AVAILABLE, LAY IT FLAT ON THE TABLECLOTH OR TOWEL.) TO AVOID BREAKAGE, PASTA SHOULD NEVER GET TOO DRY.
- IN A LARGE POT, BRING FOUR QUARTS OF WATER, AND A TABLESPOON OF SALT TO A BOIL.
- ADD PASTA AND COOK FOR 5-7 MINUTES ONLY, CONSTANTLY STIRRING TO AVOID STICKING.
- DRAIN, SERVE, AND

ENJOY

NONNA'S TRADITIONAL MARINARA SAUCE
SERVES 4

1 12-OUNCE CAN CRUSHED TOMATOES
1/4 CUP OLIVE OIL (NONNA PREFERS VIRGIN)
1 LARGE CLOVE GARLIC, MINCED (ADD MORE IF DESIRED)
1 TEASPOON FRESH OR DRIED PARSLEY (NONNA PREFERS FRESH)
1 TEASPOON CHOPPED BASIL
1 TEASPOON SALT
A PINCH BLACK PEPPER

✛

- IN A LARGE SAUCEPAN HEAT OIL.
- ADD GARLIC AND SAUTÉ ON LOW FLAME UNTIL GOLDEN.
- ADD CRUSHED TOMATOES, PARSLEY, BASIL, SALT, AND PEPPER. COOK ON LOW FLAME FOR ABOUT 45 MINUTES, FREQUENTLY STIRRING TO AVOID STICKING. IF SAUCE APPEARS TO STICK, ADD HALF A CUP OF WATER.

KITCHEN MEMORIES

BY SHOBHA SHARMA

I see Amma cooking on the mud washed stove
Over red coals making hot *sambhar,*
With small red onions.
I enjoy the familiar odor, but stand far away shy and nervous,
Having lived with her mother for six months.
Amma has a beckoning smile
And I slowly inch towards her,
Calling her "Maami" instead of "Amma."
Years later she says she thought she had lost me forever.

I see Appa sitting on the small stool
Eating his meal at eight in the morning.
He is impatient, late for work.
Soundlessly, Amma serves him,
The steam rises over rice
And colored plastic spice containers dance in the sunlight.

It is winter in wartime and we ration rice.
Amma makes *chapattis* and
Yellow *dhal* with green cilantro.
The *nei* is marbled white stone
And sticks to the spoon stubbornly.
We sit on mats and wait for the kerosene stove to melt it.

Amma and Appa find coconuts in the new house.
There is coconut chutney with *dosai* now.
Amma teaches me to cook; she is very strict and says
I should know the difference between golden brown and burnt.
I grind the *masala*, moving cylindrical stone on rectangle;
Back and forth, back and forth.
She warns, "Watch out, do not put your finger there,
Look out, let it not spill over."
I learn to carefully collect and wash the stones.

Amma has changed and so has her kitchen.
She has a marbled counter top,
Gas stoves and electric blenders.
The stones, kerosene and coal stoves are gone,
But we still ooh and aah as she mixes and grinds
And simmers and creates wonder in her kitchen.

PICKING BLUEBERRIES

BY BILL SHERWONIT

he stains on my pants are steadily growing in both number and size. Spreading and overlapping, they now form an archipelago of dark, rounded islands on the tan nylon sea that covers my legs. The color of deep muscle bruises on the mend, these bluish-purple blotches come from the bodily juices of squashed blueberry fruits, which I've been hunting in the mountains east of my Anchorage home. The stains are most abundant around my right knee, reflecting my habit of kneeling on it when my lower back begins to ache from too much bending over.

Pants stains are a crude measure of my success at finding local berry crops. Lots of stains, lots of ripe blueberries. Of course, I have other, more dependable ways of documenting success: most obviously, the number of quarts I collect or the number of pies and berry pancake breakfasts that my picking yields. Yet there are more subtle measures, too: the stiffness in my back after hours spent hunched over ground-hugging tundra bushes; the joy of discovering a rich "new" patch that other berry pickers have ignored or overlooked; the invigorating pleasure of inhaling crisp mountain air while caressed by warm August sunlight and serenaded by redpolls or sparrows.

Though a half-century old, I am new to berry harvesting. Certainly I've picked and gobbled these tiny wild fruits for as long as I can remember, whenever walks have taken me through berry patches. But only in recent years has such casual picking become a more formal seasonal ritual. Now, in late summer and early fall, I sometimes head into the backcountry expressly to collect wild berries. Even in this northern climate, the variety of edible types is remarkable: salmonberries, watermelon berries, high- and low-bush cranberries, nagoonberries, gooseberries, cloudberries, crowberries, huckleberries, strawberries, raspberries, ligonberries. Blueberries have become my favorite target, because of both their taste and widespread abundance; they're everywhere, it seems, from Alaska's lush coastal rain forests to high alpine meadows and expansive arctic tundra.

I try to recall what caused the shift to serious collecting. Gradually, the memory takes shape: in the mid-1990s, while exploring

Alaska's wild coast, I'd stumbled across an incredible profusion of juicily delicious blueberries. The last day of the trip, I filled two quart-sized water bottles with purple-blue fruits larger than peas and brought them home to share with Dulcy, my wife. We gobbled fresh blueberries, then blueberries with milk, and, finally, I tossed blueberries in pancake batter. Forever hooked by my experiments in berry pancakes, I asked Mom (a most excellent baker) for pie recipes. Her easy-to-follow, step-by-step instructions deepened our berry delight. And so I became a berry gatherer.

In just a few years, this harvesting has evolved into a valued ritual. In Alaska, where summers seem too short and autumns are even shorter, berry picking is one way to celebrate the changing seasons, instead of fighting the downhill slide into winter's cold and darkness. It's also a way of becoming better acquainted – and more physically connected – with my home landscape. As a berry picker, I pay more attention to the places where I walk. I learn about plant associations and the conditions that produce blueberry bushes, notice changes in the timing and quantity of ripened berries from one year to the next.

One place I inevitably check is aptly named Blueberry Hill, a gently rounded knob in the Chugach Mountains a few miles from home. A short walk from the trailhead, the hill is an invigorating place of high winds, alpine meadows, and grand views that take in much of south-central Alaska. Kneeling on Blueberry Hill's pale brown soil, crawling among yellow, orange, and reddish-purple bushes and grabbing berries one by one or in small bunches, I can't help but become more grounded in the local landscape. And by collecting and consuming the berries that grow in my wild "back yard," I more fully participate in the seasonal cycles; I digest and absorb the fruits of my homeland.

Last year, my best harvest ever, I picked three gallons of blueberries. This year, surprised by an early ripening and faced with smaller "crops" in my favorite picking spots, it's likely I'll gather only two gallons, maybe less, by autumn's end. A tiny haul by most harvesting standards. And hardly worth mentioning, when compared to the bulk fruits and vegetables and meats (and junk food) that Dulcy and I will purchase at the grocery store this year. So in one sense, I suppose, my picking is a token effort. In another sense – and the way I choose to see it – my harvest is a symbolic act, a personal reminder that *all* my food comes from the earth, not from supermarkets and food-packaging producers. Just as these wildly delicious berries from nearby mountains feed my body, so the act of picking them feeds my spirit.

ODE ON A BEET

BY VIVIAN C. SHIPLEY

All ye need to know
– John Keats

Boil raw beets for the pleasure
of it, the old way of it, the work of it,
curly green leaves whistling
to bloody veins. Sunflowers race
for sky, untrellised peas languish,
but beets survive shade of cucumber
too nearly planted. Into yoga, beets

don't fight for space, compete
with zucchini. Beet nubs heave,
grow, big or tiny, fissure at the neck.
Large beets peel naturally, small beets
are reluctant, not ripe. Breens steamed,
nubs boiled, cold garnet liquid saved
for dye; wanting this world to be
enough, I leave a taste of dirt, of earth.

A WOMAN CAN LIVE BY BREAD ALONE

BY VIVIAN C. SHIPLEY

I get it all from earth my daily bread
– Tony Harrison

Imagine, me in England. The White Crusty,
the Cut and the Uncut. The Small Tin,
the Large Tin, the Bloomer. A cottage loaf,
round, white and bouncy like feather pillows,

down filled mattresses and if the topknot
is missing, I'll be teething a farmer's loaf
dusted with flour. If I finger square corners,
four by eight inches, brown, light, smooth,

not grainy, I will know for sure it's Hovis.
Ciabatta and *briôche* found their way
across the English Channel. So can I.
For a change of pace, picture me in India.

Let's say Bombay for the caption. I will stuff
chapatti, phulka so hot it burns my tongue,
tandoori nan and the even sweeter Frontier
version, *Peshawari nan,* in my mouth all at once.

Overloaded? Not until I eat *reshmi roti,*
the *shirmal,* the *paratha* will I have the need
to compensate for the sin of over indulgence.
Simplify, me in Karachi, Pakistan. No servant.

Backdropped by dawn, I wait in line for a loaf
outside the Monastery of the Angel's stone wall.
Baked by the nuns to honor God, the bread is
rationed as if there were a war. No bulk buying.

Stuffed with money, my pockets will be emptied
for a few bites of crust. A hatch opens. My head
must be bowed, my eyes averted while I file
past, right hand extended as if I were a sinner

sticking out her tongue for communion's grace.
A wooden tray slides out with my allotted bread,
white, soft, light like the wings of an angel surely
will be, floating me to what heaven can be had.

COOKING LESSONS

BY KAREN KOWALSKI SINGER

ust before Easter, I get a call from Debbie. "Do you want me to teach you to make matzoh balls?" She knows I love them. Ever since I got my first taste at a Passover Seder she'd hosted at our church a few years ago, Debbie always makes sure I get a margarine tub filled with matzoh balls in her rich homemade chicken broth whenever she makes them. But she only makes matzoh balls at Passover, and I told her once that if I knew how to make them, I could have them whenever I wanted. I'm like a kid, wanting my birthday to come every day.

"Yes," I say, knowing that as much as I want to, in reality I am required by friendship to do this, even if I didn't want to, even if I have to give up a Saturday morning's sleep and my private quiet time. This is the first Passover since her mother's death six weeks ago, and the first Easter since my mother's death last September. Deb needs me to be there to watch and learn and to share a ritual activity, and I need to participate, because our mothers are no longer with us and we feel like orphans. She has no mother to pass judgment on this year's matzoh balls.

Deb has invited my family: Tom, Carrie, Emily and me, to the family Seder on Saturday night, and my dad, too. And she's invited her mother-in-law and one or two work friends. She checks with me about each addition to the guest list, telling me, "It's *our* Seder," meaning hers and mine. I don't disagree with her on this point, but I know this is what she needs to do for herself, to move through her grief. As she chatters on about her mother's matzoh balls and family holidays of her childhood, I wonder if she's headed for a fall — can these matzoh balls possibly be good enough?

"The perfect matzoh ball," she begins as we sip Bavarian chocolate coffee before beginning to cook (the lecture first, then the lab), "Let me put it this way: there are two schools of thought about matzoh balls. There's the fluffy school and the hard and chewy school. The Epstein family belongs to the fluffy school."

She sets me up at the kitchen counter, mixing eggs and matzoh meal and water with my fingers. I feel like a kid making a mud pie. If my nose gets an itch, I'll be a matzoh mess. She tells me the secret of the fluffy matzoh ball – adding the margarine last, in little chunks, not melted, as the recipe on the box recommends. The margarine melts as it cooks, leaving little air pockets resulting in fluffiness. We drink more coffee while the dough chills in the fridge. Fifteen minutes, not one second more or less. We pull up little pieces of dough and roll them into gritty balls between our palms. She keeps checking mine for size.

Then they are ready to go into the boiling water. They must cook for 45 minutes, which seems like an awfully long time to me. I'm amazed at her patience with this process – I know I'd be pulling them out of the water to check every few minutes. This is the way it's done. We sit down for more coffee and more talk, this time doing that catching up we need to do, comparing our grieving. Since I am six months ahead of her in grief lessons, I listen and am able to give tips and pointers – yes, I experienced that; yes, that gets better. The dreams, the images that catch you unawares when you think you might get through a few hours without picturing a gurgling tube, hearing a moan or rebuking cry – it does diminish, I tell her. But also, I say, nothing will ever be the same in your life again. You have no mother, and you have to be the mother to yourself.

She begins to tell me her family stories, her family's unique way of being Jewish in Skokie, Illinois. It makes me think about my family, and what we have that we can call "tradition."

◇ ◇ ◇

We weren't particularly big on tradition in our family. The fifties and sixties weren't the era of diversity, but of the melting pot. I didn't like being of Polish descent. The children at William Howard Taft Elementary School told jokes about dumb Polacks. There were many Polish people in Detroit, whole neighborhoods of babushka ladies and men with bulbous noses and shapeless jackets. There was a whole page of Kowalskis in the Detroit phone book that my brother sat on when he outgrew his high chair. And there was the Kowalski Sausage Company, no relation to us, but a mean boy named Dennis teased me, calling me Karen Kowalski Hot Dog. Polacks were stupid, spoke English with that thick puddingy accent: they were men who smelled of musty old age, women with babushkas hooding their foreheads. We saw them on streets in Detroit, where my grandparents lived, and at the little shop where Dad stopped to buy *kasha* and mushrooms, but never in Wyandotte, our little suburb, new and fresh and American.

The newly built midwestern town my all-American family lived in was a suburb of Detroit. Rows of small uniform houses lined the streets. Inside the tiny starter home at 1269 Tenth Street, we sat on blonde wood chairs, drew back curtains printed with 1950's Miro patterns, set our cups on Danish modern coffee tables. I never thought of myself as anything but American.

But I knew my grandparents were Polish immigrants. When we drove into the city on Sunday afternoon, through Hamtramck, through the tunnels and concrete, to Davison Avenue where my paternal grandparents lived, or River Rouge, were my mother's family was, we entered an older world. Things looked different, and the smells — potatoes, dill, mushrooms, old buildings and old people, perfume and must, the bakery and the buses — my nostrils were alert to each rich, dark and complex scent.

And the foods we were served at either Grandma's house were different from what we got at home — *kielbasa*, polish sausage, *kishke*, sauerkraut, mushrooms. Most of it didn't suit my Wonder Bread taste. I would have preferred the macaroni and cheese my mother made, or ring baloney fried with onions, my personal favorite. Our meals at home were the Good Housekeeping variety, with bread and smothered round steak, mashed potatoes and canned green beans, or spaghetti made with tomato soup sauce. But my mother had a few Polish dishes she prepared, which were popular with the entire family: stuffed cabbage made in the pressure cooker, and *pierogi*, the noodle-like dumplings filled with rich chopped meat and onions, and served with melted butter sauce. She also made them filled with tangy sauerkraut, but the kids would gorge themselves on the meat-filled ones, leaving the sauerkraut for the adults, who inexplicably, seemed to like it.

We even liked the word, the way my parents pronounced it — which we could barely duplicate. The rolled "r" stopped on our tongues. "Pya-duggi." We'd try again and again to roll it in our mouths.

Pierogi were so much work to make, they were only for special occasions. The first thing my mother had to do was cook a huge roast, the kind of dinner we would have only on Sunday afternoons, maybe when we were having company. There had to be plenty of leftovers. The next day she'd rummage in the cupboard for the meat grinder, a contraption that she'd clamp to the Formica dining room table's edge. The meat pieces would be pressed into the funnel at the top, and then Mom would press down the meat while she turned the handle smoothly and quickly, watching the ropes of cooked ground meat falling in loops into the bowl.

Sometimes my brother Lee and I would ask to turn the handle, but it was hard work. We couldn't do it too many times before giving up, wandering out into the living room to play Tinker Toy city or watch cartoons, but only after sneaking a bite of that cold roast beef.

Then she would make the dough. On the large wooden breadboard, she'd measure out a mound of flour and salt and with her fingers make a hole in the top of the mountain. Cracking two eggs into the well and adding some water, she'd then begin mixing the egg and water into the flour with a knife. Some of the liquid would escape, and she'd catch it with the edge of the knife, flipping it back into the flour. Soon it had become a raggedy dough, and she'd start to knead it. The egg-y dough stuck to her fingers, looking like raggy bandages. If the phone rang in the middle of this process, someone else would have to answer and hold the phone to her ear. She'd add more flour, kneading and turning until the dough was smooth and dimply. My job was to get a heavy bowl from the cupboard and run hot water in it for a few minutes, then pour out the water, and wipe it dry. The bowl, now pleasantly warmed, was popped over the dough resting on the board. It needed 10 minutes, she told me. Why? Because why.

When she'd mixed the filling − meat, browned onions, a little salt and pepper and a dollop of sour cream to moisten − it was time to make the *pierogi*.

The sharp knife sliced through the dough ball, leaving an edge, exposing the inside, cratery and rough, though the outside now was smooth and soft, white and dusty with flour. Snick-snick, cut in half, then quarters, then each quarter cut in thirds and each third cut in two pieces − 24 little blobs of dough in all. I'd get to roll the blobs into balls between my palms and Mom would roll out each ball into a circle with the red-handled rolling pin. Then, cradling the stretched dough circle in her hand, she added a spoonful of meat mixture in the center and deftly flipped the edge over into a half circle, crimping the edge with her fingers. They always looked perfect, perfectly shaped little pillows resting on the wax-papered plate.

A big blue spotted roaster was filled with water, placed over two burners, and brought to a boil. Then she'd slide the dumplings into the water a few at a time, cooking them until they floated to the top. Then they were placed in a bowl and drizzled with melted butter. How could we wait until dinner to taste them?

This was the food I craved when I grew up and went away to college. When I talked to my mother on the phone before a visit, I'd ask, "Will you make *pierogi?*" On one of those trips home she told me if I wanted them I'd have to make them, and she put me to work so I could learn the technique hands-on. Anyone could tell which ones she had rolled and which were mine – lopsided, too thin in some spots, too fat in others, the crimps either too wide and scallopy or so narrow that they'd split while cooking, spilling meat and sauerkraut into the pot. It was more than a cooking lesson. It was tradition, something you must be taught, something you learn by practice, something of my ancestry to carry on, something I'd one day want to teach my own children.

My brother Mike loved *pierogi* and when he came home on leave from the Army, he didn't ask, he just expected Mom would make them. He liked them so much that when he married, he sent his wife to Mom to learn how to make them. My sister-in-law, another Debbie, was so painfully shy and quiet that my sister and brother and I all had a hard time getting to know her. Conversations with her had to be jump-started and might die a few times before we'd give up and turn back to each other, teasing in our usual acerbic way. The conversation would have passed her by. I dreaded telephone conversations with her, dreaded the dangly silences when I ran out of questions to ask her. But she and Mom had something in common, and Mom was her champion. Maybe what they shared was a troubled childhood, or a difficulty with self-esteem. When my sister and I griped about our frustration with one-sided conversations, Mom always defended Debbie, and we felt rightly chastised.

When we were planning the memorial service for my mother, ordering the meat and cheese trays and relishes and veggies, I called my sister. "We really should have *pierogis*," I said, "but I don't have time to make them."

"Let's ask Debbie," she said.

They were the tenderest *peirogis* and the most savory I have ever tasted. She and Mike had made the dough and stuffed the dumplings with beef and cheese and potatoes, but brought them uncooked from their home two hours away. At our house after the service, they boiled the water and stood at my stove with a slotted spoon, lifting out the white dumplings while we waited, mouths watering.

My mother's half sister Judy, whom I hadn't seen in 20 years, and her half brother Dennis had come from Michigan for the service. Judy said to Debbie, "How do you get them so tender?" Her husband Mitch teased, "Yes, tell her. Judy's are never this good." I looked at Debbie's face and got a glimpse of how a group of people grow into a family.

Sitting around the freshly polished table, in a room filled with flowers and green plants we'd brought from the church after the service, we talked and laughed and reminisced until it was time for Judy, Dennis, and Mitch to leave for their home in Michigan. Somehow those *pierogis* had transformed the meal into a joyful sacrament of shared history.

◇ ◇ ◇

Debbie splits the last of the chocolate-y coffee between our cups, and starts a new pot. Her kitchen windows are misted with steam from the boiling kettle. A wholesome smell surrounds us of matzoh and butter and boiling dumplings. Debbie inhales the scent. "It smells just like my mother's kitchen."

We could almost believe we're in a Polish village kitchen a hundred years ago, if not for the ticking of the kitchen timer and the drip of the electric coffeemaker.

When the timer rings, it is time to taste test the matzoh balls. With a slotted spoon, my friend Debbie dips one out into a bowl and cuts it in half. Her first bite she offers to the sky. "What do you think, Ma?" and *"Mazeltov!"*

Then she looks at me. "Well, what do you think?"

I take a bite, blowing on it a bit so I won't burn my lips. It's tender, fluffy and wonderful.

"Perfection," I say.

THE WAY TO A MAN'S HEART

BY GRAZINA SMITH

rank Merriman mopped the beads of sweat that peppered his forehead and called, "Honey, I'm home!" He walked toward the kitchen and asked "What's my little Candy made for supper today?" Frank was winded from climbing the five steps on the front porch and puffed as he entered the room. Candice flipped her perfect blonde pageboy with her long red fingernails. *He's early. Traffic must be light,* she thought as she glanced at the clock. *Maybe it's my cooking that makes him hurry home.* That possibility creased her lips into a smile, but the smile never softened the glint in her blue eyes.

As she stirred the soup, Candice glanced up at Frank and recited the menu. "I made wild mushroom soup, marinated avocado salad, prime rib roast, twice baked potatoes, and fresh green beans. The beans are flavored with bits of smoked bacon, just the way you like them. There's also hot, home-made bread with sweet butter. For dessert, I made butter-crumb apple pie and vanilla ice cream." She turned and gazed at Frank. "I was lucky to find the vanilla beans, or you would've had to have strawberry."

Candice watched Frank closely as she described the feast and waited for his approval. She didn't flinch as he leaned over to peek into the pots, and the odor of his sweat mingled in her nostrils with the tantalizing aroma of food. They didn't have a shower and Frank had not bathed for more than two weeks. As he gained weight, he found it increasingly difficult to climb in and out of their high, old-fashioned, claw-footed bath tub. Candice never nagged about his personal hygiene. As a matter of fact, in their four years of marriage, she had made few demands. Candice beamed when Frank kissed her on the cheek.

"Candy, honey, I was so lucky when I found you. All the men I know are jealous. They can't believe that girls like you are still around to marry." He laughed. "At noon, people stare in amazement when I unpack my lunch."

Frank's mouth salivated at the memory of the three thick, Virginia-baked ham-on-rye sandwiches she had packed for him today. Swiss cheese provided a mellow counterpoint to the smoky ham, and a pint of dill-mayonnaise potato salad complemented the sandwich. Everyone around him gaped when he took out the plastic container of blueberry buckle dessert. It was full of berries wrapped in a crust and swimming in rich dollops of whipped cream. Frank rubbed his chin in memory of the juice that had trickled down there.

Candice began to bring the food out to the dining room. She always set the dining room table and today a cobalt blue pitcher, filled with daisies, stood in the center. Her blue willow patterned china contrasted well with the dark red placemats. Crisp white linen napkins, folded into a bishop's miter, stood guard above the forks. She quickly arranged the platters of food, working them like a jigsaw puzzle, until not an inch of the table was left uncovered.

From their first days together, Candice prepared wonderful meals and made sure they were not eaten in front of the TV. She wanted Frank to realize meal time was a special occasion and very important to her. After dinner, he often spent the night in front of the television, drinking beer and eating his fried pork rinds, and that was all right with her, too.

Frank tucked his napkin under his chin and began to stir the hot mushroom soup. This wasn't the pale canned variety but a rich chestnut brown in color. As he dipped his spoon, bits of carrots and potatoes danced to the surface. He could see three varieties of mushrooms: the plump white oyster, European brown *crimini* with their distinctive dark caps, and the delicate *shiitake*, all floating in the velvety broth. Frank inhaled the savory steam as he brought a spoonful to his mouth and, to do the soup justice, he had a second helping. Then he cut a two-inch thick slice of prime rib, pale pink and fork-tender, marbled to perfection.

Early in his relationship with Candice, Frank noticed that his enjoyment of food gave her great pleasure. Nothing he craved to eat was too much effort for Candice to prepare. He assumed all this was a tangible expression of her love. Frank's appetite expanded until recently it had become indiscriminate. During the day, he snacked on store-bought cupcakes, potato chips, and candy bars with as much relish as the meals Candice spent hours preparing.

Truthfully, he sometimes enjoyed the junk food more. At home, Candice seemed to count each mouthful he took. Although everything was delicious, he sometimes felt that he ate to satisfy a hunger in Candice, perhaps a need to justify her efforts in the kitchen. It looked as if she measured each forkful and used it as an assurance of Frank's love for her. Frank glanced at Candice's plate. She was squeezing a bit of fresh lemon on her salad. A small portion of broiled sole rested next to it. "Oh Candy, Candy, how can you eat like that with all this wonderful food around you?" He sighed, secretly admiring her restraint.

Candice smiled. *How strange,* she thought, *both of my two previous husbands gave me the same nickname.* Of course, her name did lend itself to that diminutive. Frank knew she had been married once before, but not twice. Candice's mother had told her that it was proper to keep some secrets in a marriage.

Harry, her first husband, was truly greedy. He took no notice of her or what she ate. He was always pleasing himself, stuffing himself, and never offered her a kind work or a bite to supplement her salads, but after all, it was his greed that had attracted her to him. Her second husband, Paul, was a little more considerate, but his concern was always voiced with a regretful, "Oh well, this really isn't good for you," as he rammed food into his own mouth. At least Frank commented on her meager meals; however, he never seriously tried to dissuade her from her perpetual dieting. She suspected he took pride in her slim appearance, feeling somehow that her shape enhanced his worth.

She straightened her size eight dress and answered, "Don't worry, Frank. I love cooking for you. It makes me happy to see you enjoy the food I make; and besides, my mother always said the way to a man's heart is through his stomach."

Frank cut another slab of meat and speared a second double baked potato, oozing with cheese.

"I mixed the sour cream and fresh chives myself. Have a little more," Candice coaxed in a little girl voice as she nudged the dish nearer to him. "Tomorrow I thought I would make duck á l'orange. Why fry chicken when you can have duck?" She raised her long lashes and smiled across the table.

Frank looked up and a gasp escaped his throat. He hunched forward and began to claw at the red checked shirt that covered the broad expanse of his chest. He turned to Candice, made a choking sound and toppled over, his cheek smacking into the slice of prime rib on his plate. Candice watched with a frown on her forehead. Soon she could see the blue tinge around his lips. As it became more pronounced, his complexion turned pale and waxy. Candice got up slowly, walked over to Frank and delicately felt the artery in his neck. It appeared to be still. Should she call the paramedics now? She wondered. Candice knew it would not do to wait too long, but she wanted to be sure. After all, she'd worked hard for his estate and his insurance. However, would a third husband dying of a heart attack arouse suspicion?

"Oh, but that's ridiculous!" Candice whispered to herself. What she had done was not illegal and a long time ago, she had convinced herself that it was not even immoral. After all, Candice had given each man exactly what he wanted: a thin, compliant wife and all the rich food he could eat. She was patient, always finding the right victim and setting no timetable for her ultimate goal. She encouraged their weight gain and never complained about her marriage, knowing her skills in the kitchen would eventually free her and be her current husband's undoing.

Candice dialed 911 and began to sniffle into the phone. Soon she was crying copiously, and the operator made her repeat the address twice. When she hung up, she wondered if Frank's life insurance, his stocks, and the sale of the house, would provide enough money to finally open the restaurant she'd always wanted to own. She had money from her previous marriages, saved in a secret bank account, but she'd had to use some of it to finance her latest "cookacide." Frank had been frugal and insisted on a budget. In the past year, the budget had became tighter then ever. However, Frank had been naive enough to accept her explanation that she bought all his rich, exotic food on sale. He assumed that he had married a poor but clever widow who was a superb cook. He had not been entirely wrong and Candice did not begrudge spending some of her savings. Her mother had always told her, "Nothing ventured, nothing gained," and she considered the money an investment that would bring a good future return.

With Frank's death, she expected to have enough to finally open her restaurant, or at least have sufficient collateral to qualify for a substantial loan from the bank. She knew good restaurants were expensive to run and they often took two or three years to show a profit.

An ambulance siren, drawing nearer, broke into her thoughts. She glanced at Frank. His head lay on a pink pillow of meat. She shivered at the fat congealing on his plate. Four years was a long time to avoid eating almost everything she cooked. She did two hours of vigorous aerobics every afternoon, just to burn off the small portions she tasted to correct the seasonings. Candice knew her body was an important outer package of a total product she had to sell and she was glad she would not have to go through this charade again. Thoughts of her sacrifices and subterfuges gave some honesty to her tears.

The paramedics were kind to her, but there was nothing they could do for Frank. She cried helplessly, automatically making sure that her eyes were not puffy and her nose did not run. Candice noticed the older man eyeing her butter-crumb apple pie. A glance to his left hand assured her that he had no wedding ring. Her mother had taught her to always keep her options open, and Candice remembered everything her mother said.

A week later, she sat in Lawyer Barnes' office waiting to find out the full extent of Frank's estate. She watched the thin, colorless man aimlessly shuffle papers on his desk, moving them from one stack to another. He had asked for coffee, and they both sat waiting for his secretary to bring some. His sparse, dull red hair was plastered over his bald spot in careful lines like rusted tracks in an abandoned railroad yard. Candice amused herself by imagining Lawyer Barnes positioning the strands each morning, overlapping them on his rounded pink dome. She controlled her smile as she imagined him pasting each strand down with some sort of super glue. It took her a moment to realize that Lawyer Barnes was speaking to her.

"Mrs. Merriman," he mumbled again as he sat on the edge of his chair. "I guess we should get down to business, however unpleasant."

"Yes." Candice said and dabbed her eyes. She crossed her legs, slightly hiking her skirt, and gave him her full attention.

"You know that with Frank's current difficulties, there isn't much left for you. Of course, the house has only a small mortgage," he quickly added.

One glance at her soft mouth, open in a round "O," made him realize that she knew little about Frank's financial problems.

"Current difficulties," she repeated. For a moment, Candice thought the man was speaking a foreign language and her brain could not decipher the words.

"Well, he had made some bad investments about two years ago in the stock market. Lost a lot. That was compounded by the loss of his job nine months ago."

"Unemployed?" She gave a little strangled gasp. "But he went to work every day."

"He was embarrassed to tell you, although I advised him otherwise. He was always hoping he would find something soon. In good weather, he spent a lot of time in the park; when it was cold or raining, he went to the movies, the library, or visited me in the office. We were good friends." The lawyer shook his head sadly. "It was his obesity, you know. The company claimed it kept him from doing his job. They gave him warnings and some time for compliance. I told him we might have legal recourse, but he couldn't make up his mind. All he seemed to be able to do was eat. I don't know how a man can let himself go like that."

"But his life insurance?" Candice was grasping at straws.

"Canceled. That was all job related, you know."

Sam Barnes handed her a mug of coffee. He wondered if taking her to lunch would soften the blow. *She's an attractive woman,* he thought. *It's a shame Frank hasn't provided for her.*

Candice noticed that he took three heaping spoonfuls of the dry creamer and six large spoons of sugar in his coffee. She always observed such details. Her mind was already weighing the merits of a food-loving paramedic versus an unattractive, but hopefully greedy, lawyer as a future mate.

EGGPLANT

BY LISA SORNBERGER

You grow out of a flower,
slip into your own skin,
purple as midnight's silk horizon,
the way that sunset
transforms itself into night.
You are the way
land embraces light,
the perfect curve of melding
heaven and earth,
union of spirit and skin.

Suspended from a tenuous stem,
you touch and taste the earth,
reminding us that our birthright
is to delight, to shine,
to be unafraid of being flesh.
You are as purple as acted-on passion,
heady as grapes ripened to full readiness,
Eve's gift in September's garden.

LEFTOVERS

BY RICHARD STELLA

The tomatoes have gone flat
the celery is brown
the mushrooms are black and green
and the cheese is fuzzy.

The milk is way past its
      use-by date.
I smell it anyway and put it back,
next to the green tuna casserole
you brought me and wonder
why we don't date anymore.
Thanks for the Pyrex.

Sometimes it's best to start from scratch.
Don't take home leftovers I know
      I'll never eat,
realize that wine doesn't last as long as milk
      at least at my house,
and promise not to hold on past the
expiration date and

next time I cook for a lady
      I think we'll go out.

THE UNSPEAKABLE WEIGHT OF EMPTY

BY BEVERLY SWEET, R.N.

growing small as
thin air she is
her own disease
 a dwindling girl
numbs mounting pain with
vice clenched teeth while
sorrow seeps from
a sleeve of skin and
vacant
child
empties

15 year-old

diagnosis: depression with psychotic features
            anorexia

ORIGINAL SIZE

BY BEVERLY SWEET, R.N.

Some pictures make it look as if Eve wore a size 6.
I wonder if she did. I wonder if Adam would have expected more
for the precious price of a rib?

What if Eve wore a 16? Would it have mattered to the snake?
Do you think he would have gone all slack-jawed and ended up
forked-tongue-tied?
Or maybe he'd just relax and lose the mean streak?

What if he had?

My bet is we'd all still be sitting there in that
big old lush garden with everybody getting mail at
the same address
and about a-kazillion relatives
might be killing time in a chat room at
www.thisisallthereis.com

What if Eve wore an 18? Or a 24?
What in heaven's name does any of that mean, anyway?

Just for fun let's imagine Adam coming home from another
long day hanging with the Lord to find his
little woman trying on leaves,
all because silly old Satan
let the C-A-T
out of the B-A-G
and Eve got embarrassed by
all that nakedness and flesh...

Wow.
If Eve was full-figured

I guess she'd dump size fig
to try to squeeze into
size
banana.

THE PRODIGAL FEAST

BY CLAUDIA VAN GERVEN

Forgiveness, for all its niceties,
is a slippery business. Take the fatted
calf, for instance, or indeed,
the entire feast. Was it pure
generosity, unequivocal acceptance?
I mean, why have a feast at all?
Why invite all the neighbors and the resentful
son? What could such a gesture signify?
What could all those thin slices of veal
declare when the old man slipped them
tenderly on the boy's plate? Who could help
but remember the desertion, the debauchery
when the indulgent father
ladled thick gravy over sliced
muscle? And what could all those exquisite
baby peas summon up for the wastrel
but an abacus on which to number
his degenerate days, his arrogance, his mis-
calculations? What could that public pudding be –
no matter how many cupsful of sugar –
but a bitter paste with which to stick
the errant boy in his place? Resentment is
a delicate sauce. It lasts forever. He would never
wash the grease of that lenient meal
from his shriven face, never quite digest
the shame of that succulent supper.

MEMORIES FROM THE HEARTH

(ANIELA PITENSKA KONIOR, 1893–1995)

BY DIANALEE VELIE

he sweet, warm aroma of baking *babkas* always filled the house as I was growing up; always, it will remind me of my grandmother and her large, strong, able hands. Strong, patient hands that kneaded our bread, cooked and cleaned, and loved and lasted, showed us our own hands could tackle any job from baking bread to building bridges. When my hands have been strong and busy, it is her hands I have seen. She has taught me, with her own calm strength, not to fear the unknown. Her hands guide me always on the rails of life's bridges; bridges I can build and cross. My own hands inherit her intensity. I know I can do.

We grew up on the *babkas* Babci made in Brooklyn. *Babkas*, warm and fresh from the oven, we ate with gusto. We toasted stale thick slices and spread them with jam. Staler still, those slices became breadcrumbs for cooking. Any leftovers, we gave happily to the birds. My memory flies, like those birds, to a fire escape in Brooklyn and to the *babka* crumbs I held out in my hands as a toddler. Now, in the woods near my New Hampshire home, this legacy has followed me, securing a tender place in my heart as I replenish my bird feeders and scatter my own *babka* crumbs on the ground.

I often wonder who taught my Babci to cook. My mom and I learned without ever knowing, watching and helping her, then baking *babkas* on our own. Love rose within us like the yeast of our dough. Babci taught us without ever trying. I can't help but wonder who taught her to cook and I can't help but wonder who taught her to love. I am sure neither came easily. When her own mother died in Poland, her father remarried a woman with other daughters. My family's own little cinder tale began there. Unwanted and alone at eight years old, little Aniela was put on a ship. America became her promised port of call, her final destination the home of an aunt and uncle she had never met in a city of unknowns in an unknown world. Good-byes, I am sure, were in her heart. Good-byes to the farm she loved and the horse she thought was her own. In Massachusetts, at work in a garment factory all day, her hands learned to use a needle and thread. Did she go home to help cook the meals? Is it there she learned to knead those *babkas* or did the memory come from the ache in her heart for her missing mother? Is there a cookbook written in the soul? Did they love her dearly here in America or tolerate her as a family burden? Whenever I tried diplomatically to ask her, she only shrugged and said with a smile, "Life is beautiful when you are being busy being."

At 14 she met my grandfather and started to sew her own wedding gown. At 16 she married him and my family was founded and headed for Brooklyn. The timid smile on her face in her wedding photograph is not the strong self-assured smile to which I grew so accustomed. But her hands are the same. They are the hands of a doer. They are the strong and capable hands my mother, daughter, and I possess. We are doers and we can do. We know how to bake Babci's *babkas* and we know we can do whatever else life calls upon us to do. Babci's memory continues to restore my soul. Up until the day of her death, at 102 years old, she still called me her Dinusha, a diminutive Polish nickname that somehow makes me feel taller. My strong hands have assured her Babci's *babkas* are here to stay. They are a gift, a legacy, of simple strength.

When that sweet warm aroma fills my own kitchen, my family, friends and neighbors know that Polish bread is in the oven. *Babka* can be served with breakfast, lunch, or dinner; better yet, this same recipe can be rolled thin and filled with cinnamon and sugar, poppyseeds or prunes, for a sumptuous dessert. See which you like best, and remember to save the last precious crumbs for the birds.

BABCI'S BABKAS

2 PACKAGES OF DRY YEAST

1 QUART OF WHOLE MILK

1/2 POUND OF SWEET BUTTER

1 CUP OF SUGAR

1 POUND OF RAISINS (1 BOX)

1 AND 1/2 TABLESPOONS OF SALT

5 EGGS

3 AND 1/2 POUNDS OF FLOUR (14 CUPS)

MIX 2 PACKAGES OF YEAST IN 1/4 CUP OF WARM WATER TO WHICH ABOUT A TABLESPOON OF SUGAR HAS BEEN ADDED.

WHILE THIS MIXTURE IS RISING, SCALD THE QUART OF MILK AND MELT THE BUTTER IN IT. SLOWLY STIR IN THE SUGAR.

WHEN THE MIXTURE IS LUKEWARM, ADD THE YEAST MIX, SALT, AND RAISINS.

BEAT FOUR EGGS AND STIR IN SLOWLY, ALTERNATING WITH THE FLOUR.

KNEAD THE DOUGH UNTIL IT COMES AWAY FROM THE SIDE OF THE BOWL.

LET RISE UNTIL THE DOUGH DOUBLES.

PUNCH DOWN, PUT INTO LOAF PANS OR PLACE ROUNDED ON COOKIE SHEETS AND LET RISE AGAIN FOR HALF AN HOUR.

BRUSH THE TOPS WITH A MIXTURE OF ONE EGG AND A TABLESPOON OF MILK.

BAKE AT 400 DEGREES FOR THE FIRST 10 MINUTES AND THEN LOWER THE OVEN TO 350 DEGREES AND BAKE FOR 30 MINUTES MORE.

ENJOY!

BAKING BISCOTTI

BY DIANALEE VELIE

Baking *biscotti,*
strufoli, perringoza,
Italian cookies sweeten
my disposition
in the making.
But today hunger
invades my kitchen,
following me to my study
where I must write
about this need
to create cookies,
this hunger
that drives
me to write and bake,
this need, saying
feed me,
I am starving.

Feed me
and I will acclaim
that which cannot be attained
in words or stanzas,
in cookies or in sweets.
Working
in flour or in ink,
at my computer
or by my sink,
on blank page
or empty baking sheet,
my appetite affirming
the metaphor of methods
by which I master my muse
and worship
the consuming desire,
the adoration of process,
that makes
me complete.

SUNNY SIDE UP
BY KEVIN WATSON

ll I wanted was a hot breakfast. I'd been on the road since six o'clock the previous evening, having left straight from my brokerage office in Denver. I didn't even take the time to change out of my business suit. The two-hour drive to the Kansas state line wasn't bad, but the six hours across Kansas was brutal. I fought the urge to sleep while creeping along Interstate 70 at 70 miles an hour. Of course, I could have fallen asleep at the wheel and, chances are, never left the road. I-70 stretches across Kansas like a yardstick on a kitchen table, and at night it's just as exciting. But I had to reach central Missouri by 7 AM for the state auction of my Uncle Henry and Aunt Shirley's farm. Low-interest government farm loans, government-controlled crop prices and a few droughts finally did them in. I was there to offer my support and help them bid on a few items they wanted to keep in the family.

My last visit to Morgan Grove was 12 years ago, for Uncle Henry and Aunt Shirley's 25th wedding anniversary. I told myself for years that I was going to come back to trout fish the Gasconade with my uncle, but a volatile market and my more volatile marriage always made me put it off until the next year, then the next.

My partners had taken to shouting at every little Wall Street hiccup, and my wife had taken to doing the same every time her attorney suggested that my attorney and I were both trying to screw her, which, as I told her, would be very difficult since someone else was already doing her the honor.

I really needed a breather, and drove just so no one could track me down and demand I catch the next plane back to Denver. I even tossed the cell phone into the trunk.

As Uncle Henry would say, I was "hungry as a farm-raised trout" when I pulled into Morgan Grove just before six in the morning. Main Street rolled through town like a long welcome mat. The small shops, even the bank, seemed to bow politely, welcoming me as I drove past. The only soil out of place was on the cars and trucks parked in front of Sandy's Three Squares Diner at the other end of town.

When I stepped into Sandy's, the aroma of frying bacon and brewing coffee turned the gnawing in my stomach up a notch. The smell of smoldering cigarettes was even tolerable.

I took the first stool at the counter next to an elderly gentleman in overalls, nodding a "hello" to him before fixing my eyes on the wall menu above the coffee machine.

A middle-aged waitress with broad hips and sassy eyes plopped a coffee cup down in front of me. "You passing through, sweetie, or just come here to rescue me from all these rednecks?"

"Drove in for the Maynard auction," I said.

She raised an eyebrow. "So what'll it be?"

"Three eggs, sunny side up, crisp bacon, wheat toast and coffee."

She hollered my order back to the kitchen then turned away without another word. I spent the next minute soaking up the ambiance — the pickled eggs in the two-gallon jar next to the manual cash register, the gold-speckled Formica walls, the early morning risers, mostly farmers, lining the counter and filling the booths.

The waitress returned to fill my cup three-quarters full with the last bit of coffee from a glass pot. I raised the cup to my lips and blew on it for a few seconds before taking a sip. It was strong and very cold. I waved the waitress back over.

"What'cha need, darlin'?"

"My coffee is cold," I told her.

She glanced down at my cup. "Well, you're just going to have to drink it a little faster now, aren't you?" She grabbed a steaming pot from the hot plate behind her and filled the remaining quarter-cup. "There you go. Nice and warm." She then filled the cup of the gentleman sitting next to me. "Your plate'll be right up, Walter."

"Excuse me," I said, gaining her attention again. "You think I could get another cup of coffee?"

"To go?" she said.

I raised my cup. "Another cup. A hot cup?"

"Why, you haven't even drank that one yet." She chuckled and moved on down the counter offering more hot refills.

The cook, an old man with arms flailing like he was trying to put out several fires, tossed a plate up on the order window, and yelled out, "Walter up!"

The waitress scooped up the plate and delivered it to the man next to me. "There you go, sugar. I'll be right back with the jelly."

"Fed up!" called the cook.

The waitress took this order and dropped it in front of me without a word. The eggs were scrambled, the bacon was limp and greasy, and the toast was charred beyond recognition. I think it was white bread, not wheat. I studied the fare delivered to Walter. His eggs were perfect, his bacon crisp, his toast tanned and buttered. I prodded my eggs with my finger. They were rubbery and cold.

"Miss?" I waved the waitress over again.

"You can't be ready for your check," she said. "You ain't even touched your food yet."

"This isn't my order."

Just then a man at the other end of the counter called out: "Hey, Eunice, you think I can get my breakfast before lunch?"

Eunice fired back: "Keep your pants on, Carl! Lord knows all the other men do when you're around." She turned back to me. "You ordered your eggs sunny side up, right?"

"And my bacon crisp," I added. "And wheat toast, a little less done."

She picked up a slice of charred toast and grimaced. "Is kind of overdone, ain't it?"

"And the eggs are cold," I added.

She winked at me. "I'll take care of this." She tossed the plate back up onto the order window, and shouted, "Blake, these eggs are cold!"

Blake shot back: "Well, they wasn't when I cooked 'em!"

"Three sunny side, crisp bacon, and wheat," Eunice hollered. "Get it right this time." She smiled sweetly. "Just be a minute, honey. How's your coffee?"

"It's... fine." I took a sip and nodded my approval, in spite of it tasting as if it could strip the chrome off a bumper.

As soon as Eunice was out of earshot, I directed a question to Walter, who was enjoying his hot, well-cooked breakfast. "There another diner around here?"

He nodded while he chewed, then said, "Got a Pancake House in Rolla."

Rolla was another hour's drive south. "I mean around here, close by."

Walter sopped up some egg yolk with his toast. "Nope."

When I was a boy, having breakfast at the Three Squares with Uncle Henry was a favorite part of our early morning fishing trips. We would sit at the counter, just like Walter and I were now, drinking coffee, mine with extra cream and sugar, Uncle Henry's black and strong, the way I drink mine now. Back then the small café would be filled with farmers in oil-stained caps, dusty overalls and cake-dried boots. They were rugged men, educated by experience. Political lines would be drawn and then immediately crossed. They were a joking lot, tossing around insults like they were sowing wheat. The only sacred ground was family. Tell a man his wheat crop was looking good, knowing full well that he's got 400 acres of corn he's about to harvest, but not a word about the wife and kids, unless you're asking if they're well. These same men would rub my short brown hair and wish me luck on their way out, each carrying with them the sharp scent of their farms, a mix of hay, motor oil and manure.

I looked around and could see that these men had changed. They were no longer boisterous and opinionated. They seemed withdrawn, even suspicious, like men who had come to doubt even the rain.

"Sunny side up is up!" shouted Blake. "Crispy bacon, wheat toast! I miss anything?"

"Only a good education and the last train out of town," Eunice said, scooping the plate up and whipping it over in true waitress fashion.

This time the wheat bread was lightly toasted, and the bacon crisp. The eggs were cooked to perfection, sunny side up, overlapping in the middle of the plate. And topping off the eggs was an inch-long cigarette ash.

I dropped my head onto the heels of my hands and rubbed my eyes, wondering if I had actually fallen asleep at the wheel, crashed my car into a telephone pole and was now paying for all my transgressions.

"Everything okay, sweetie?"

I raised my head and opened my bleary eyes. "My eggs."

"What about your eggs?" Eunice asked.

I counted to three and exhaled slowly. "There is something on them."

"You don't want pepper on your eggs?" she asked.

"That's not —"I caught myself before I exploded. "— Not pepper."

Eunice took a closer look. "Walter, what's this look like to you?"

Walter gave my plate a glance. "Pepper," he said.

I slipped my fork under the ash and carefully lifted it off my eggs. "This is pepper?"

Eunice, wrinkled her nose. "It does look kind of suspicious."

"Suspiciously like a cigarette ash?" I asked.

"Or from one of them skinny cigars people smoke these days."

I placed the ash-laden fork back on the eggs and nudged the plate toward her. "I don't mean to trouble you, but this seems to be the only diner within 60 miles of here." I pointed to Walter's plate. "If I could just get what he's got so I don't have to trouble my Aunt Shirley to feed me before the auction..."

Eunice pressed a hand against her breastbone and she suddenly appeared ill. "Aunt Shirley?" she said.

Walter snickered. "That's what he said."

The fire came back to Eunice's eyes. "I heard what he said, Walter! Just eat your eggs and hush!"

The door opened and Eunice tossed a smile over my shoulder. "Help you, gentlemen?"

I rubbed the back of my neck; the pickled eggs next to the cash register were beginning to look tasty.

"Two coffees to go," I heard someone say.

Eunice shuffled over to the coffee: "So, you boys just passing through, or do you have a glass slipper you want me to try on?"

"We're looking for the Maynard farm. Can't seem to get good directions," someone said.

I swiveled around and found two men in business suits. I was prepared to offer directions, provided they had a bag of donuts in their car, but Walter laid a heavy hand on my shoulder and spoke first.

"You boys running the auction?"

The older of the two smiled a bit nervously. "We're just here to catalog the sale. Basic accounting, that's all."

"I'm headed that way," Walter said, leaning on my shoulder as he took to his feet. "Need a part for my tractor."

Eunice handed the two men their coffee and rang up the sale. "Ya'll be sure and stop back for lunch, ya hear?" She winked. "I still need to try on that slipper."

Walter squeezed my shoulder. "Nice meeting you, son."

As soon as Walter ambled out the door with the two state accountants, Eunice called out: "Give me three sunny side, crisp bacon, wheat toast, and no foolin' this time, Blake. This here's Shirley and Henry's nephew, for cryin' out loud."

I wheeled back around and found Eunice pouring me a fresh cup of coffee.

"I am so sorry," she said. "I thought you was one of them state fellers, you in that fancy suit and all. I feel just awful. Blake really is a fine cook. He'll have that breakfast you been craving right up. No shenanigans this time."

I looked at my watch. "How about just a sweet roll to go?"

"Sweet roll nothing, honey." Eunice patted my hand. "Just sit there and relax. That auction ain't going to start without them two state fellers, and Walter's on his way to pick up a part for his tractor. I bet they follow him half way to Rolla before they realize he ain't going nowhere near your Aunt Shirley and Uncle Henry's place."

LEAVES FALL AWAY, REVEALING RIPE PERSIMMONS

BY ANTHONY RUSSELL WHITE

Leaves have to do that, it's their part.
A quick year of greening, then gravity overwhelms them.
Cold is another kind of gravity and *Down* is its verb.
But the persimmons —
their creamy oranging is less susceptible to *Down*.
And I tell you this,
I would trade you my burnt umber,
my burnt and raw siennas,
for such power.

WHEN I WENT BACK TO
BETTY'S CAFÉ FOR LUNCH

BY ANTHONY RUSSELL WHITE

there were eleven kinds of pie,
but also a smudged blank
on the black-board over the cold case,
so there might have been more,
although I don't know what they could have been.
While I waited for my BBQ Pork sandwich
out came the eraser
and ate the last Rhubarb and Peach.
John Deere and Excel-Pork had Apple and Raisin Creme,
but they stayed on the board.
The two deputy sheriffs played scratchers
and drank coffee but skipped pie,
although they appeared to have eaten some in the past.
My plate arrived just as the eraser bit
into the last Chocolate *Mousse.*
Four waitresses bustled about, no wasted motions.
Now I began to worry about my choice of pie.
Bye-bye Banana Creme, gone to Con-Ag or Cargill.
A girl in pigtails practiced her counting
with the sugar packets. Her dad is Mr. Razorbacks.
The last Fresh Strawberry was delivered
to the ERA real estate lady.
Delicious BBQ, but the iced tea is instant.
No more Pecan or Coconut Creme.
I flag down Irene and order Custard.
Safe at last.

THE QUEEN BEE

BY TAMMY WILSON

hirley dipped one finger into the banana pudding and smiled until she caught her sister's stare.

"I declare!" Iris slapped her dish rag into a sink of wilting suds. "Who'll want to eat that after your fingers have glommed over it?"

Shirley, the younger of the two, lowered her eyes to the kitchen table as if to pray. "Well, I made it! I reckon I can taste it if I want to!"

"Taste it? Lord, you nearly ate half of it!" Iris sneered at the gouge in the creamy surface, revealing brown slices of banana scattered over a cobbled layer of wafers — fly heaven in this hot weather. "Just like some fool kid, you practically ruint it!" She gave the pudding a closer look. "Looks like you should've used lemon juice on those bananas!"

"Lemon juice?"

Shirley had never been the sharpest knife in the drawer, Iris thought, but when it came to cooking, she wondered how she kept from poisoning herself or starving to death. Her sister might have been Mama's favorite, but when it came to learning how to cook, Shirley had failed the course.

"Don't you know you're supposed to dip fruit in lemon juice to keep it from turning brown?" Iris said.

"Bananas turn dark. That's their nature," Shirley replied.

"Not in my pudding, they don't!"

"But lemon juice is sour. It'll spoil the whole thing."

"OK, if you're happy with brown bananas, go ahead." Iris handed her a spoon. "Here, take this and smooth it over."

Shirley gave her sister a sheepish glance as she leveled the surface, replaced the plastic cover and slid the dish into the refrigerator next to her bowl of fruit she had brought for the family reunion. "It'll keep good and cool in there," she said.

"A far cry cooler than out here," Iris shook her head and clicked her tongue. "Banana pudding!" The thought was nauseating. She could see it now — insects with wilted wings embedded in that yellow cream! Not that she could ever enjoy such a dessert herself; she had doctor's orders about that. "In this heat, it won't be fit to eat after it sits out all afternoon," Iris said. "You'd have thought Crystal would have asked for something you can leave out, like pound cake or coconut cake."

Crystal was the new "waitress," wife of their brother Raymond and Iris's least favorite in-law. Lord, she was almost young enough to be his daughter — just a hair over forty — and with twice the mouth as his first wife, Phyllis, who was now living someplace near Raleigh.

Shirley stepped over to the counter. "Coconut cake calls for dairy whipped cream. That's what Mama always said — real dairy cream and coconut milk."

Iris cast a halfhearted laugh. "Mama might have known a lot about cooking, God rest her soul, but where are you going to find coconuts around here? Just get yourself some coconut flavoring and slosh some of that into regular vanilla icing. It tastes as good as any real coconut milk and it's a lot cheaper."

As soon as she'd said it, she wished she'd never given away her secret; now Shirley would probably blab it all over town.

"Is that what you do? Cheat on your recipes?" Shirley said. There was a tartness in her voice.

"Come again?"

"Crystal said she only wants family recipes for the reunion, so you can't cheat with shortcuts," Shirley said.

"Well, of all people, she should know about cheating, stepping out on her first husband to take up with Raymond!"

"Now Iris, don't you go into that!"

Crystal and Raymond's romance had grown on the county grapevine months before the two of them finally got married. That had been nearly three years ago, with the middle-aged Crystal in white lace and rhinestones, playing the part of the blushing bride, standing there in one of those Gatlinburg wedding chapels! She had plenty to blush about, too. That paunchy Raymond was no prize, at least not the last time Iris had seen him — a thin wing of hair combed over his bald spot and belly flopped out like bread dough without a pan. Mama would turn over in her grave seeing how he had turned out.

"Don't forget it takes two to tango. Besides, Raymond was stepping out on Phyllis and he is our brother," Shirley said.

"Don't remind me." Iris wiped the counter with hard swirls.

"He said Crystal's a better cook than Phyllis, so at least she's got that going for her."

There was no doubt their brother had been eating well, Iris thought, but he had always been heavyset.

Shirley scratched her head, covered with bobbed gray hair straight as pine needles. "Anyway, Crystal was put in charge of the reunion. She knows what goes with what, since she worked at the Highway Café." She pronounced café as if she knew French, like the actresses Iris had seen on the soaps.

"Waiting tables? That's hardly the same as being head chef!"

"They don't have a chef down there. They just got them regular cooks."

"Well, I'll leave my cooking to me, and Miss Crystal can just tend to her own affairs," Iris sniffed. "Who does she think she is, the Queen Bee?"

Shirley folded her arms across her chest as she stared Iris down. "The fact is, you just don't like her!"

"That's right," Iris rattled a bowl onto the drain board. "I have never have cared for upstarts who pretend to be something they ain't. It's one thing for her to take over the reunion, but now she's dictating to all of us what to bring."

"The reason she's in charge is that she's organized. Somebody has to see to it that we don't all bring the same thing."

Iris glowered at her sister. It was just like her to not stop and think things through. She had always been that way, even back when they were kids. Shirley would get her feelings hurt, then run to Mama every whip stitch. Mama would always back her up, too, just because she was the youngest and prettiest, never wearing hand-me-downs like the older children. Not Shirley! Mama would scrape together enough egg money to buy material to make her new clothes. One time, she had spent a whole two dollars on one of the *real* Shirley Temple dresses in the Sears & Roebuck, only to see that brat drip gravy all over the front of it the very first time she wore it to the family reunion. That was back before they had the likes of Crystal running the show. It made Iris sick the way her own sister was sticking up for that floozy.

"Bring the same thing! Fat chance of that!" Iris said. "You ask a bunch of us Funderburks to a do, we have enough sense to bring something besides dessert."

"Well, then, what *are* you bringing?" Shirley opened the refrigerator door. "You got potato salad made up?"

"No."

"Then what you got?"

Iris swished silverware into the tepid water. "Nothing."

"You can't bring *nothing!* What are you going to do when they have the recipe swap?"

"I reckon they'll have to skip over me."

Shirley's eyebrows arched higher. "But that's the best part! Everybody stands around and tells about their dish and how they learnt to make it."

"I guess Crystal will have to do mine, then," Iris said crisply.

"What?"

Iris put her hands on her aproned hips and thrust dripping forks at her. "You couldn't pay me to take a jar of chow chow to that reunion!"

Shirley's jaw dropped. "But *everybody's* going! Crystal said the whole family's invited, in-laws, outlaws, everybody!"

"Then count me with the outlaws! All I hear's what *Crystal* says!"

"Well, she asked me to bring that banana pudding, so that's what I'm doing," Shirley said.

Iris felt as hot as a radish that had been left in the ground too long. "Good for you! You just go and enjoy your banana pudding and Crystal and all the rest of them! Just leave me out of it!"

"What if they ask where you are?"

"You tell them my sugar's acting up. Besides, they all know I don't have no business eating all that stuff," Iris said.

"But that's not the truth."

"Is so."

Shirley's brown eyes flashed dark olive. "Well, it sounds like you put your problem with Crystal ahead of the rest of us!"

"If I have to include the likes of *her* in the family, then I guess you're right! That floozy with her hair all piled up like some bee's nest and all that makeup makes her look cheaper than she is, and that's about as low-rent as it gets." Iris punctuated the air with her index finger.

"She's not *that* bad!"

"Bad? She's nothing but trailer trash!"

Shirley's lips formed a firm line. "Raymond doesn't live in no trailer. Besides, I wear makeup and that don't make me trash!"

"It don't help none."

"Well! If that's the way you feel, I have a notion to take my banana pudding and leave!"

"Well, why don't you do that?"

"Well, I think I just might!" Their eyes locked for a few seconds before Shirley swung the refrigerator door open and jerked the pudding dish off the shelf, nearly rattling a jar of pickles to the linoleum.

"I hope the *Queen Bee* chokes on it!" Iris said.

Shirley wheeled around holding the pudding between them, her cheeks as flushed as a ripened peach. "Iris Funderburk! That's the most un-Christian thing I've ever heard you say!"

"I'm just telling the truth. I haven't seen either of them warm a pew in over a year. Tell *me* what's Christian!"

Iris steadied herself on the counter, her eyes blazed. She knew better than to get so riled, but how dare her own sister stick up for that tramp!

"Sounds like you need more medication," Shirley snapped.

"Oh sure! Bring *that* up like I'm some drug addict!"

"Iris, you always get this way when your sugar's acting up!"

"Oh I do, do I? Well, you just take your old pudding and get yourself over to the Legion Hall and tell the Queen Bee and the rest of her *family* to have a nice time!"

◇ ◇ ◇

It was a good thing the table stood between them. She could slap Shirley, she was so angry, just like the time Mama had forced her sister's hair into Shirley Temple ringlets and then let the little darling play at Iris's vanity. The four-year-old had spilled powder and nail polish, all worth good money Iris had earned selling peaches, then had taken a bottle of cologne and sprayed it the wrong way into her eyes. The child, by then a screaming terror, had wailed like she'd been swarmed by a nest of yellow jackets.

"Iris! You're older! You need to look out for your little sister. You know she can't resist temptation!"

Mama's words had stung like the preacher's on a Sunday morning. Later, Iris had "looked out" for her little sister all right, playing keep-away with what few things she had worth keeping away, like her diary. Shirley had found it one day and Iris had wrestled it away from her, and on cue, she had run off bawling to Mama. Other times, Shirley had goaded Raymond into teasing Iris about some boyfriend, or threatening to break her toilet water bottles, or even hanging her underthings on the front porch; the two of them would squeal with delight.

One time Iris's date showed up as her hosiery and panties flapped over the banister, tied to a thin line of rope. It had been Raymond's doing with Shirley's help, of course.

"I don't know what's to become of y'all," Mama had said. "Raymond, you ought to be ashamed of yourself."

Shirley got off scot-free, as usual. Eventually she grew up to marry and raise a family, with plenty of help from Mama, who, coming down with the rheumatoid, became Iris's responsibility. She waited on the ailing woman hand and foot until the day she died.

◊ ◊ ◊

Now a wrinkled, baggy version of the bratty, mop-topped tyke stood before Iris. "Have a nice time? This is your family, Iris! I never heard of the like," she said.

"Well, you have now!"

That's when Iris stuck her tongue out. She hadn't exactly meant to do it, but she'd done it before she could stop herself.

Shirley drew back like a shocked kitten dipped in water. "Why Mama was right! You are nothing but a big old baby!"

"And you're still a brat!"

Shirley huffed, her lip quivering before she turned heel and slammed the door, rattling dishes in the cupboards. In the wake, Iris stood like a stunned deer for a few seconds before she steadied herself to the kitchen table and sat down. She swatted at a fly as the room warped around her. She felt like she was on a silent rowboat about to tip over. Things were going to go black real quick if she didn't find a piece of fruit, a cup of juice. She must have something sweet right away!

In a cold sweat, she leaned to open the refrigerator door and peered around the milk and orange juice. On a lower shelf sat an unfamiliar bowl, the plastic kind made to look like cut crystal. Shirley must have left it in her hurry, and now there it sat, full of cool cubed pears, peaches, grapes and bananas, already rounding out and ready to turn brown.

Iris sat the cold dish in front of her and hesitated as the room rode out another wave. Then she hungrily dipped her spoon into the bowl of proffered salvation and closed her eyes.

ANOTHER WHITE MEAT

BY DAN WITTE

I n a small, dimly lit restaurant on the north side of Moline, where diners could request a window table offering a slightly impaired view of the Mississippi – or, on quarter beer nights, a substantially impaired view of the Mississippi – Harmon Nunn stared at the plywood Carp-O-Meter hung alongside the salad bar and felt an angry gas bubble carom through his intestines. For one thing, the Carpettes were late, and he couldn't help thinking that it might have something to do with a contentious encounter he'd had with the lead singer's breasts two nights earlier, at the conclusion of an otherwise pleasant evening spent regaling her with tales of his entrepreneurial heroics while plying a melodic little Bordeaux he'd just added to his wine list. Somehow – he couldn't really remember how – as he was standing behind her to help her put on her coat, he'd inadvertently wrapped his arms around her, and then inadvertently cupped her breasts in his hands, and though he'd made it abundantly clear that he was merely attempting to maintain his balance, the singer yelped as if she'd been shot and brought a dish of complimentary butter mints crashing onto his head.

There was also the fact that the carp itself hadn't yet arrived – or maybe it had, but was possibly misplaced somewhere; it was hard to say for sure because his day manager, who he'd just that morning put on a tips-only basis, had stormed out a couple of hours earlier, and the remaining staff didn't speak English. This was a disturbing development in that the carp was the central feature of the weekend's CarpFest, set to begin in just a few hours, and of course the very reason for the Carp-O-Meter and the scheduled appearance by the now tardy Carpettes.

Doubly frustrating for Harmon Nunn was that the carp was coming from Americarp, a little fish farm he himself had opened on the boggy Mississippi floodplain a year earlier. Having had the good fortune to sell his estranged wife's shares in typewriters.com before the tech stock crash, he subsequently threw the windfall at an entrepreneurial impulse that visited him like a distant, conniving relative. Hadn't Americans shown an interest in so-called "traditional" American cuisine? Hadn't they embraced meatloaf and mashed potatoes, and, more importantly, the previously maligned catfish? Conditions couldn't be better for the ascendance of another despised bottom dweller, he thought, and he adopted what he hoped would become a hallmark advertising pitch: "Carp: Another White Meat." That he hadn't sold a single fish over the ensuing year, that he'd failed to stoke the culinary imaginations of restaurateurs and diners alike, that carp seemed destined to remain a fringe and rural dish, like rabbit and squirrel – while it can be debated whether these realizations had coalesced so literally and rationally in his mind, they were in fact the impetus for CarpFest, which he'd been desperately promoting for the preceding two weeks.

An hour before the restaurant was scheduled to open, Harmon Nunn drove to Americarp to investigate the delay, and found the dozen carp ponds seemingly emptied of fish, and his lone remaining attendant, Mercurio, vanished – which, in a different set of circumstances, might have been a relief. How many times had he come here and watched the fat brown fish roll in their fetid water, their pectoral fins breaking the surface like lazy, malfunctioning periscopes, their stupid gelatinous eyes searching for the odd bug or fecal debris, and wished that a piscine plague would come along and kill them all?

Now, however, as he walked quickly from pond to pond throwing in bread crusts – which would ordinarily provoke a swarm of greedy, sucking carp, but which now sat idly on the surface until they became waterlogged and sank – the apparent dearth of inventory prompted a vague sense of panic, accompanied by audible and mildly painful tremors in his digestive tract. Calling out his attendant's name, he walked to the garage, and though most everything seemed to be in order, he had a nagging sense that something was missing, something that had been so permanent a fixture that he'd probably ceased noticing it. As he got into his car and pulled out onto River Drive, the thing that was missing sped past him in the other direction: Americarp's delivery truck. And while he had only a second or so to look as it passed him, two things occurred to him: first, it was headed in the wrong direction, away from him and his restaurant; and second, didn't it look like there were three people crowding the cab?

◇ ◇ ◇

Antonio Almonte wanted to be called The Toenail. Most people instead just called him Tony, or occasionally Tony A, which he viewed as being too pedestrian, lacking the kind of mysterious, comradely respect conferred on certain of his associates, such as The Hammer, The Shark and The Iceman, but he wasn't really sure how one went about setting up one's own nickname. Should he begin referring to himself in the third person? Maybe use certain forms of "persuasion" in order to encourage the use of a particular nickname? But, really, did one even get to choose one's own nickname? Wouldn't it, almost by necessity, be a name that others bestowed upon him?

Thinking about his nickname was something he did when he was avoiding thinking about other things. Right now, for example, one of the things he didn't want to think about was his faltering business, Skin n' Bones Pet Food, Inc., whose slow-selling product lines included Can O' Gristle for dogs and Can O' Mouse for cats. He was troubled by the public's general disinterest in these brands, and by some recent inquiries from the Health Department regarding his ingredients. Another thing he didn't want to think about was the new product line he was preparing to debut, in part because he feared it would stall like his other products.

The idea had been proposed by the night watchman he'd recently hired, whose name he always had a hard time remembering – Marcuso or Mercurium or something like that. After a shift change one morning he'd handed Tony an empty can with a mock-up label.

"So, what do you think?" the guy said.

"Can O' Crap?" Tony said.

"Can O' what?" the guy said.

"That's what I'm askin'," Tony said. "What're ya doin' calling my stuff a can o' crap?"

"Wait, gimme that," the guy said, and he frowned as he looked at it. "No, no, see, you're reading it wrong; it says Can O' Carp," and he tapped each word on the label as he said it. "See? Can-O'-Carp."

And so this Mercury guy, or whatever his name was, promised he could deliver a ton of carp, on the premise of splitting any profits fifty-fifty with Skin n' Bones Pet Food.

"No risk to you," the guy said confidently, reassuringly.

"So, what, you're a commercial fisherman?" Tony said. "Got a boat on the river or what?"

"A boat on the river," the guy said. "Yeah. Yeah, I got a boat on the river."

Although intrigued by the idea, Tony was nonetheless uneasy about the carp itself. This Mercado guy, or whatever his name was, just didn't seem like the fisherman type – which, in itself, wasn't a problem. The gristle, after all, was sourced through a disgruntled sausage plant employee, and the mice through some kids working in the junior college science lab. But the fact that it was being delivered on a Saturday evening, of all times, seemed a little bit too...what was the word? Amateurish? Was that even a word?

He thought about that word: amateurish. He said it out loud a few times, the dull acoustics of his wood paneled office flattening his voice. "Amateurish," he said. "Amateurish, amateurish." It sounded made up, he thought, like a make-believe nationality or religion, which made him think about the origins of certain words – carp, for instance, who ever thought of the name carp? – which brought him back to The Toenail. He said the name out loud, then started testing it in sentences – "Hey, heard about The Toenail?" "Hey, The Toenail ain't going to be happy about this" – when he heard the rumble of a truck backing into his cargo bay. He put on his windbreaker and briefly considered his reflection in a framed motivational poster. Did he look like The Toenail? Maybe that was the problem. Maybe he didn't look like The Toenail. But wait – who could really say what The Toenail should look like? Wouldn't he, by virtue of being the first Toenail, define what The Toenail looked like?

These were his thoughts as he walked into the cargo bay, where he saw a white cloud of exhaust dispersing amid the faint smell of burnt oil, three people climbing out of the truck's cab, and the big garage door slowly descending. And just before the door closed completely, just as the last of the three people stepped down out of the truck – his night watchman, it looked like, but who were the others? – he heard the squeal of rubber outside his cargo bay, and saw a blue sedan with tinted windows. Great, he thought, the cops. And then someone shrieked. It might have been the woman, but Tony would have sworn it was that Mercury guy.

◇ ◇ ◇

Jittery yet largely sedentary, overwrought and overweight, Mercurio Jones was an almost perfect candidate for a heart attack. In fact, when he thought about his death – and he thought about it constantly, contemplating with stupefied horror the complete cessation of consciousness, the utter vacuum of nonexistence – he imagined it would be an epic coronary event, each of his arteries seizing like a kinked garden hose as he frantically tore out great curling swaths of his chest hair.

He'd known anxiety all his life. As a child he'd been called hyper and high-strung, and in high school, uptight. His stomach was perpetually clenched like a fist, his bowels fluttered like a flag, and if he occasionally flew off the handle and into a fit of rage, and beat somebody senseless in the process, it was because he was excitable, maybe even hysterical, and people should have just known better.

Downshifting as he approached the Rock Island city limits, his eyes darted from one side view mirror to the other, expecting to see a swarm of flashing lights bearing down on the stolen truck. Why had he agreed to this plan? It had made him nervous from the start, since he'd first been approached by Harmon's wife and the dude from the restaurant – both of whom sat alongside him in the cab now doing nothing, which agitated him. It was their plan; they were the ones who'd brought him the classified ad for the night watchman job at Skin n' Bones. It would be easy, they said. Get in there, get to know the owner, and make him an offer. If he pulled it off, and the guy agreed to the fifty-fifty split, they'd give Mercurio half of their share. And God knew he needed the money. Minimum wage didn't go very far, even in the Quad Cities.

Now, as he rumbled up to the loading dock at Skin n' Bones, and began backing into the cargo bay, he allowed himself just the faintest glimmer of optimism. If he could just get inside, get the carp unloaded and into the rendering and pulverizing machines – hissing and thundering contraptions whose intake manifolds sat churning inside pits excavated in the factory's concrete floor – if they could just pulverize and can the evidence, and get the truck back to Americarp, how could anyone ever prove where it had come from?

Before he'd cut the engine, Harmon's wife and the dude from the restaurant were already climbing down out of the cab, which made Mercurio even more nervous because he hadn't told Mr. Almonte he was bringing anybody along. He'd wanted to get out first, see Mr. Almonte, make a few introductions. Now, however, as he stepped to the ground and glanced out toward the street, as the big garage door slowly rolled down, a car came skidding to a halt on the apron, and Mercurio felt something tighten in his chest. He heard a noise, a kind of terrified falsetto screech, and was surprised to discover that it came from him.

Panic like an electrical current convulsed his muscles, and then he was running, just running...running somewhere, anywhere, he wasn't sure where, his legs feeling as if they might become detached, his lungs swallowing sheets of molten air. He heard voices behind him, urgent, disembodied, vaguely familiar voices possibly getting closer, and so he turned to look behind him as he ran, and he saw the dude from the restaurant, and then Harmon's wife, and then Harmon himself, and even Mr. Almonte, and they were all running and waving their arms, and they were saying something to him, something that he couldn't quite make out, something about the floor, or no, wait, something about the, the...what? The something, the...the...the machines, that's what they were saying, the machines, something about the machines, and they seemed to be yelling louder, but he was running faster, opening more distance between him and his pursuers, when he felt the floor disappear from beneath his feet, and felt himself momentarily suspended in the air as if there were suddenly no gravity, as if he were one of those Saturday morning cartoon characters running off of a cliff.

Then he was falling, the law of gravity suddenly, cruelly reinstated, and he felt the toes of his shoes slip between the rolling wheels of the pulverizing machine, and heard the sounds of snapping and crunching. He felt a sense of absolute, brilliant clarity as the first wave of pain shot up through his legs, and though his impulse was to yell, he felt strangely out of breath, out of air, as if he were submerged in one of the ponds at the fish farm, and then it seemed as if the machinery stopped, even as he felt himself being pulled further into the great rollers. There was no sound, no feeling, no smell or taste; he could only see, and what he saw, a hundred yards away and yet as close as if he were standing right there, was the injection line, and an endless single-file procession of cans waiting to be filled. He wanted to read the labels on the cans, but now his sight began to fade, so that the last thing he was aware of seeing were just a couple of words: Can O'. And now, simultaneously descending and ascendant, he felt he didn't need to read the label at all, he knew exactly what it said. Can O' Mercurio. He was sure of it, and it seemed in some way fitting, and he marveled at the ingenuity of it.

HOLD THE ONION

BY MARGARET YOUNG

It is the size of your fist.

It is not round
the way the Earth is not.

Its crust scales, puckers dryly
in colors of skin and stone.
It smells of enclosure, endings.

Under a long earthquake crack the flesh
is slick and green.
This is how the onion breathes.
Stripped bare
it will pant, shrivel, and fade.

Brown veins connect the poles,
gathered and cut paper twist
to tangled mat of root
like a dry squashed spider,
a wire moustache pressed
into an eyeless face.

If Cinderella's coach had been made from an onion
it wouldn't have stopped at the palace
but rolled on into the night
trailing streamers of iridescent crepe
copper spokes glinting
the moon squinting
bitten
out of the ashblack sky.

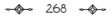

WATERMELON

BY MARGARET YOUNG

Any way you slice
it smiles, tender white
or hard black teeth
askew, gritty pink
spit sticking hands that slip
grasping a chin of rind:
lift its mouth to yours,
kiss, drink.

TWINKIE DREAMS

BY PEGGY ZABICKI

omorrow is the first day of my two-week vacation and my fabulous new diet. This is the best diet in the world because I feel like I will really succeed this time. I can eat whatever I want, in any quantities, anytime, but – yes, I have a but. My but is that you can eat whatever you want but you have to eat everything standing naked in front of a full-length mirror.

Monday, Day 1 – This morning I ate two bites of corn flakes. My eyes kept focusing on the pouch of skin hanging just below my waist and a bit over my pubic area. The corn flakes seemed to go directly there. It was like trying to eat while watching surgery. I washed the two bites down with coffee, got dressed and mopped the kitchen floor. I felt slim and light. By 10:30 AM I was starving, so I got undressed and made a low fat bologna sandwich with cholesterol free mayonnaise on extra fiber diet bread. I wolfed down the first bite but the second one I had trouble with. It stuck in my throat. I shouldn't have been looking at my saddle bag thighs. Dinner I don't want to talk about. Who can eat spaghetti naked?

Tuesday, Day 2 – This morning I had a headache and felt very hungry. What a wonderfully productive way to spend my vacation. Feeling proud of myself, I marched my naked body right in front of the mirror clutching a toasted bagel with cream cheese. I was able to eat almost the whole thing by taking large bites and focusing on my toes. My glance up to the fat deposits on my inner thighs prevented me from finishing, though. I worked at the computer until lunch. The land of WordPerfect was replaced with a microwave burrito. I rushed to the mirror with my lunch, leaving a trail of clothes behind me.

One problem with eating and standing is where do you put your napkin? I found that I could keep it handy by lifting up my left breast and tucking the napkin under there. It worked out so well that I forgot it was there until I discovered it at my 3 PM snack. Standing like Eve herself, I ate an entire apple before discovering the forgotten napkin. After the apple I got dressed, read the mail, saw an old box of valentine candy on the table by my bed, got undressed, ate three chocolates, got dressed

Wednesday, Day 3 – I seem to do best when eating foods that don't need chewing. I was able to swallow a whole bowl of instant Cream of Wheat with a pat of diet margarine easier than say, scrambled EggBeaters or instant breakfast bars. Watching myself chew brings that familiar lump to my throat. I decided to have ice cream for lunch.

Well, that Cream of Wheat and ice cream really gave me energy! While I was planning dinner, I accomplished so much. I spent all morning at the computer, and then I vacuumed rugs, scrubbed the bathtub, did two loads of laundry and made lots of phone calls. I called my best friend, Cecelia, to tell her about this great diet. At 5'4' and about 165 pounds, she could stand to lose some weight herself, so I thought she might want to join me with this.

Why is Cecelia so contrary? So sarcastic? Laughing at me is so unsupportive. She asked me who I was dieting for – myself, my girl friends, or my current boyfriend, Raymond. I guess I'm doing it for all three. I'll feel better, I'll be a good example to my girl friends and Raymond will be pleased. I'll look better to him. Cecelia said that is a stupid reason for dieting. I don't know what's wrong with wanting to please the man in your life.

"Is he obsessing over food to please you?" Cecelia said. Well, I'm not obsessing. Cecelia asked if this means our lunch date is off. I told her that for her information I can have all the water and black coffee I want. So there. She said, get this – "Oh good, I was afraid you were going to bring your full-length mirror with you and take your clothes off in the restaurant!" Very funny. She actually said I was cranky. That stupid, moronic, ugly, idiotic bitch. I hate her. Nice best friend. I'm going to have supper early tonight.

Thursday, Day 4 – This morning I decided to take a good look in the mirror before eating breakfast. What did I see? A giant pear-shaped blob with blond hair. I tried to focus on the things I like – my ears, wrists and shoulders. That's about it. I reminded myself of a pear with caramel sauce on top. That actually sounded pretty good so I headed out to the kitchen. Cecelia called while I was reading a cookbook. She wanted to know if I was still mad. She said she was sorry. She even said she'd try to be more supportive and not laugh at me anymore. I forgave her and decided to make my famous Pears with Apricot Glaze. I cut the pears in half lengthwise as I told Cecelia about a weird dream I had the night before. I dreamt I was sleeping on a mattress that was really a giant Twinkie. Boy, I'd kill for a Twinkie right about now. Anyway, Cecelia said I'm obsessing about food and it's obviously affecting my sex life. She went on about a Twinkie being a phallic symbol. I just ignored her as I mixed together some orange juice and apricot jam in a baking dish. I then lovingly placed the pears in the pan and baked them for 25 minutes in a 350-degree oven.

Cecelia asked, "Speaking of sex, how's skinny old Raymond. Does he appreciate your new body?" I told her that Raymond actually hasn't noticed yet – it's too soon. She asked me if I thought it really matters to Raymond how big I am. I told her that I think it does matter. I wear a bigger size jeans than he does. I think he'd feel more masculine if he were bigger than me.

"When Raymond is in bed with you," Cecilia said, "do you know what his favorite part of you is?"

"What business is it of yours?" I snapped.

"His favorite part of you is – your enthusiasm," she answered.

"Oh my, you are so wise! What do you know? You don't even have a man in your life."

Cecelia said, "So what, I don't have an elephant in my life, either. Honey, don't worry so much about your so-called sex appeal. Remember, we all look the same upside down!"

Later while I was waiting for the pears to finish baking, I decided to have a nice bowl of strawberries and non-dairy whipped cream. I was already naked so I just grabbed the food and headed to the mirror. I love strawberries dipped in whipped cream, but I kept looking at my breasts for some reason. They sag a little lower each year. I believe that eventually my boobs will go so low that they'll affect my pants size.

Friday, Day 5 – Raymond came over last night with a pizza. He wanted to sit on the couch and eat and watch a movie. I told him that I was just too full to eat. I don't know if he believed me or not. He's never known me to turn down deep-dish pizza. That pig actually ate five slices. I wanted that pizza so bad I hated him. I picked a fight about something but Raymond surprised me with a gift he bought me from Victoria's Secret. I opened a little gift bag to find red and white lace thong underpants.

"Try 'em on!" he said as he stuffed pizza down his throat. I went into the bathroom and took off all my clothes in one second flat. I'm getting really good at that! Then I put on the thong. It disappeared – magically somehow – into various folds, flaps and crevices. It got sucked into all my fat! I sauntered out to the living room to model it for Raymond. He kept squinting at me and finally said, "Are you wearing it?"

I told him, "Of course I am. I remember putting it on." He did have fun looking for it. Later, as he lay snoring with pizza on his breath, I sneaked out of bed to the mirror and gobbled up the rest of the pizza. I decided to make a headband out of the thong.

Saturday, Day 6 – I set up an old card table in front of the mirror this afternoon. I can stand right next to it and put all of my food on it. It's so much easier to use a knife and fork now. This morning I'd had a heck of a time holding up that casserole dish of leftover pears. I also found that a pan of brownies gets mighty heavy as well.

This evening for supper I was feeling so light and slim that I baked a big crock of baked beans with lots of brown sugar and little slices of hot dogs. I had a slight accident, however. I was standing by the card table. I bent over that hot crock-pot and as I started wolfing down the baked beans my left nipple got burned. I just held my cold can of diet soda pop on the burn and soon it was OK. I polished off the entire crock. I'm getting used to this routine. It's great! I'm feeling thinner. For my mid-morning snack I ripped off my clothes while micowaving some popcorn. I even splurged and had a lite beer. Now that I moved the TV, I can see its reflection in the mirror. This is certainly convenient.

Sunday, Day 7 – I called Cecelia while making lunch. She asked me how the diet was going. I was putting artificial butter flakes and non-dairy sour cream on a baked potato as I triumphantly told her that I have now officially lost a total of 14 whole ounces! I asked Cecelia what she had for lunch.

She said, "I went out with Cindy and Connie and had a devil dog and cheese fries. The girls said to say hi. By the way, are you ever going to leave your house?" I told her that it just so happens, I went to the grocery store yesterday. I didn't tell her that it had been my only outing in the seven days since starting this diet. Cecelia wanted me to go to the movies with her tonight, but I told her that I would be sitting at the computer for hours catching up on some work. Besides, I thought, the expiration date on the low salt potato chips is coming up and I've got to polish those off. Then Cecelia said something strange. She said, "I love you and I miss you." Then she hung up.

Monday, Day 8 – Raymond hasn't called since the thong underpants/pizza night. I don't care. Really, I don't. I leaned on the card table and cried my eyes out while I ate a whole can of creamy deluxe chocolate frosting. Then the card table broke. I cleared it away and wheeled over my beverage cart.

I'm feeling pretty tired. I think I'll take a nap. Maybe I'll have that Twinkie dream again.

ABOUT THE AUTHORS

TIMOTHY AMSDEN
WORKED FOR THE U.S. ENVIRONMENTAL PROTECTION AGENCY FOR 25 YEARS IN KANSAS CITY, AND NOW LIVES IN THE WILDS OF NEW MEXICO, WHERE HE WRITES AND PAINTS ROCKS. HIS WORK IS IN *POTPOURRI*, *A KISS IS STILL A KISS*, AND *OUT OF LINE*, AND HE HAS PUBLISHED A VOLUME OF POEMS AND DRAWINGS CALLED *OUT OF THE BLUE*.

ELLEN WADE BEALS
OF ILLINOIS HAS WORK IN *AFTER HOURS*, *ARIEL*, *WHISKEY ISLAND*, *KEY WEST: AN ANTHOLOGY*, AND *WOMAN MADE GALLERY'S HER MARK 2002 DATEBOOK*. SHE WON THE 1999 WILLOW SPRINGS FICTION AWARD FOR HER STORY CALLED "PICKING."

DONNA BLACK
IS A CHICAGO ACTRESS PUBLISHED IN SEVERAL OF OUTRIDER PRESS' "BLACK-AND-WHITE" ANTHOLOGIES. SHE RECEIVED FIRST PRIZE IN THE *ALTERNATIVES* SHORT FICTION COMPETITION AND HAS ALSO BEEN PUBLISHED IN *KALEIDOSCOPE INK*. SHE READS HER WORK THROUGHOUT THE CHICAGO AREA.

MARGARET M. BLACKMAN
WORKS AS A CULTURAL ANTHROPOLOGIST IN THE ALASKAN ARCTIC AND AS AN ANTHROPOLOGY PROFESSOR IN NEW YORK, WHERE HER CLASSES INCLUDE FOOD AND CULTURE. HER RECENT WORK APPEARS IN *THE NORTH AMERICAN REVIEW*.

LYNNE MARTIN BOWMAN
OF GREENSBOBO, NORTH CAROLINA, HAS BEEN PUBLISHED EXTENSIVELY IN *PETROGLYPH*, *SOW'S EAR POETRY REVIEW*, *ICARUS*, *MISSISSIPPI REVIEW*, *SOUTHERN POETRY REVIEW*, *GRASSLANDS' REVIEW*, *EXPLORATIONS '99*, *THE LOUISVILLE REVIEW*, *TAR RIVER POETRY*, AND OTHERS. SHE WON THE 1998 *SONORA REVIEW* POETRY PRIZE AND HAS TWICE BEEN AN EMILY DICKINSON AWARD FINALIST.

ALYSSA BRODY
OF MINNEAPOLIS GRADUATED FROM THE UNIVERSITY OF MICHIGAN WITH A BA IN ENGLISH AND HISTORY. SHE RECEIVED HER MA IN HUMANITIES FROM THE UNIVERSITY OF CHICAGO, AND TEACHES AT CHICAGO'S COLUMBIA COLLEGE.

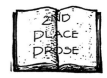

LISA BROSNAN
WRITES THAT SHE "IS RECOVERING FROM RECURRING FOOD PHOBIAS," AND THAT "A RECENT SETBACK WITH AN UNFORTUNATE BATCH OF SPLIT PEA SOUP HAS ME WONDERING HOW TO GET THAT SOUP OFF THE CEILING." THIS SELECTION IS PART OF HER UNPUBLISHED COLLECTION OF CASINO STORIES. SHE SERVES ON THE TALLGRASS BOARD OF DIRECTORS.

LINDA BROWN
WON FIRST PLACE IN FLORIDA'S 1995 FREELANCE WRITERS COMPETITION. A FORMER NASHVILLE SONGWRITER, SHE HAS POETRY IN *HAIKU HIGHLIGHTS*, *THE SAGE*, *POETRY PEDDLER*, AND *CREATIVE WOMAN*.

UTE CARSON
EMIGRATED TO AMERICA FROM GERMANY IN THE 1960S. THIS TEXAS RESIDENT PUBLISHED HER FIRST SHORT STORY IN THE 1970S AND IN THE PAST 25 YEARS, HER STORIES AND ESSAYS HAVE APPEARED IN JOURNALS, MAGAZINES, NEWSPAPERS, AND BOOKS.

MAUREEN CONNOLLY
PERFORMS HER WORK THROUGHOUT THE CHICAGO AREA. HER WRITINGS HAVE APPEARED IN *HAMMERS*, *TOMORROW*, *AFTER HOURS*, *ARIEL*, *RIVER OAK REVIEW* AND TWO PREVIOUS OUTRIDER PRESS ANTHOLOGIES.

GREG COOK

LIVES IN THE PACIFIC NORTHWEST AND HAS WORKED AS A MUSICIAN, DISHWASHER, REPORTER, TEACHER AND LIBRARY PAGE. HIS WRITING HAS APPEARED IN *ADIRONDACK LIFE*, *BLUELINE*, *HISTORY: REVIEWS OF NEW BOOKS*, AND *PARABOLA*.

MICHELE F. COOPER

OF PORTSMOUTH, RHODE ISLAND, HAS HAD POETRY PUBLISHED IN MANY LITERARY JOURNALS. THIS 2ND PLACE WINNER OF THE 1999 GALWAY KINNELL POETRY COMPETITION IS FOUNDING EDITOR OF *NEWPORT REVIEW* AND *CRONE'S NEST* LITERARY MAGAZINES.

DONNA COUSINS

HAS PUBLISHING CREDITS IN THE U.S., EUROPE AND ASIA. A FOUNDING EDITOR OF *CAREER WORLD MAGAZINE*. THIS CHICAGO WRITER HAS SHORT STORIES IN *PEREGRINE* AND *SHORT STORIES BIMONTHLY*. *LANDSCAPE* IS HER RECENTLY COMPLETED NOVEL.

CHRIS CRITTENDEN

TEACHES APPLIED ETHICS COURSES AT THE UNIVERSITY OF MAIN/MACHIAS, AND IS PUBLISHED IN *ENVIRONMENTAL ETHICS*, *JOURNAL OF BUSINESS ETHICS*, AND *WOMEN & POLITICS*.

BARBARA CROOKER

HAS POEMS PUBLISHED IN *RIVER CITY*, *YANKEE*, *RATTLE*, *WEST BRANCH*, *DENVER QUARTERLY*, *CAPRICE*, *ATLANTA REVIEW*, *PASSAGES NORTH*, *THE MACGUFFIN*, *NEGATIVE CAPABILITY*, *KARAMU*, *NIMROD*, *MADISON REVIEW*, *ROANOKE REVIEW*, AND OTHERS. SHE WON THE 2001 *BYLINE* CHAPBOOK COMPETITION.

LEE CUNNINGHAM

GREW UP IN WISCONSIN AND MOVED TO CHICAGO, WHERE SHE WORKED AS A JOURNALIST. SHE SERVES AS PUBLIC RELATIONS COORDINATOR ON THE TALLGRASS BOARD.

JOANNE DALBO

LIVES IN THE HUDSON VALLEY AREA OF NEW YORK. SHE HAS BEEN PUBLISHED IN *CHRONOGRAM* AND SEVERAL PREVIOUS OUTRIDER PRESS ANTHOLOGIES.

E.-K. DAUFIN

IS AN ALABAMA POET, PERFORMANCE ARTIST AND FAT ACCEPTANCE ACTIVIST. PROFESSOR DAUFIN HAS PERFORMED FOR UNIVERSITIES AND COMMUNITY GROUPS AROUND THE COUNTRY AND IN CANADA, BELIZE, CENTRAL AMERICA, FRANCE AND MEXICO.

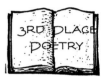

TISH DAVIDSON

PUBLISHED MAGAZINE ARTICLES ON PARENTING FOR 10 YEARS; TODAY THIS CALIFORNIAN WRITES ABOUT MEDICAL TOPICS AND HAS TWO NONFICTION BOOKS FOR MIDDLE-SCHOOLERS IN PROGRESS.

ALBERT DEGENOVA

IS A MARKETING COPYWRITER, POET, BLUES SAXOPHONIST, AND EDITOR/PUBLISHER OF *AFTER HOURS*. HE IS HALF OF THE PERFORMANCE POETRY DUO AVANTRETRO APPEARING THROUGHOUT THE CHICAGO AREA. HIS WRITING HAS APPEARED IN JOURNALS INCLUDING *OYEZ REVIEW*, *THE PATERSON LITERARY REVIEW*, *POETRY MOTEL*, *FRESH GROUND*, AND *U-DIRECT*. HIS LATEST BOOK OF POETRY AND MEMOIR IS *BACK BEAT*.

STAR DONOVAN

WAS BORN IN ENGLAND, LIVED IN SOUTH AFRICA, AND CAME TO THE U.S. IN 1984. CURRENTLY A FULL-TIME SECOND YEAR GRADUATE STUDENT IN NEW YORK STATE, SHE WRITES MEMOIRS, POETRY, AND FICTION.

CHERIE CASWELL DOST

WRITES IN CHICAGO. HER POETRY HAS APPEARED IN *AFTER HOURS*, AS WELL AS HER COLLABORATIVE PHOTO-ESSAYS WITH HER HUSBAND, HAGEN DOST.

ROBERT KLEIN ENGLER

HAS POEMS AND STORIES IN *BORDERLANDS*, *HYPHEN*, *CHRISTOPHER STREET*, *THE JAMES WHITE REVIEW*, *AMERICAN LETTERS AND COMMENTARY*, *KANSAS QUARTERLY*, AND MANY OTHER JOURNALS. THIS CHICAGO WRITER RECEIVED THE ILLINOIS ARTS COUNCIL LITERARY AWARD FOR HIS "THREE POEMS FOR KABBALAH" IN *FISH STORIES, II*.

JO LEE DIBERT-FITKO

OF MICHIGAN HAS BEEN WIDELY PUBLISHED AND IS THE RECIPIENT OF NUMEROUS AWARDS. A UNIVERSITY OF MICHIGAN GRADUATE, HER FIRST CARTOON BOOK, "...YOU NEVER ASKED FOR THIS!" HAS RECEIVED NATIONAL ATTENTION.

BARRY FRAUMAN

IS A NEW TOWN WRITERS CHICAGO GAY POET. HE HAS WRITTEN MANY EPIC AND SHORT POEMS; SOME OF THE LATTER HAVE APPEARED IN VARIOUS PUBLICATIONS, INCLUDING *OFF THE ROCKS* AND *SWELL*.

DIANNE L. FRERICHS

ENJOYS THE ADVENTUROUS LIFE OF A WANDERER WITH HER HUSBAND, GEORGE, AND DOG, GYPSY, IN A MOTOR HOME. HER FICTION HAS WON PAST OUTRIDER PRESS ANTHOLOGY AWARDS.

VINCENT F. A. GOLPHIN

OF NEW YORK STATE HAS ESSAYS AND POEMS IN A WIDE RANGE OF PUBLICATIONS INCLUDING *AFRICAN-AMERICAN CHILDREN'S ANTHOLOGY*. HIS FIRST BOOK (1999) IS *LIFE AND OTHER THINGS I KNOW*.

SUSAN HANNUS

LIVES IN A CHICAGO SUBURB WITH HER FAMILY. THIS IS HER FIRST PUBLICATION.

JULIA MORIS-HARTLEY

WAS BORN IN TANZANIA AND RAISED IN BROOKLYN. SHE EARNED AN MFA IN CREATIVE NON-FICTION FROM THE UNIVERSITY OF ARIZONA IN 2001. SHE LIVES IN TUCSON.

JULEY HARVEY

WORKS AS TELECOMMUNICATIONS SPECIALIST IN CALIFORNIA, BUT IS KEEPING HER NIGHT JOB AS PRIZE-WINNING POET. SHE CONTINUES HER SEARCH FOR THE PERFECT POET, POEM, MAN.

MARY HOWE

GREW UP IN GRINNELL, IOWA; FLORENCE, ITALY; AND MARIN COUNTY, CALIFORNIA. THIS WRITER/SPEECH LANGUAGE PATHOLOGIST LIVES IN ALBUQUERQUE WITH HER DAUGHTER.

ANNA HUSAIN

IS ASSOCIATE EDITOR OF *WHETSTONE JOURNAL* AND HAS BEEN PUBLISHED IN *PROJECTIONS* AND *MOON JOURNAL*. SHE WON 3RD PLACE IN A *WRITERS DIGEST* NATIONAL COMPETITION, 1ST PLACE IN CHICAGO'S POETS & PATRONS, AND HAS PARTICIPATED IN VARIOUS ILLINOIS POETRY EVENTS, INCLUDING READING AT BUCKTOWN ARTS FEST 2000.

SALLY JONES

OF ONTARIO, CANADA, WRITES, "IN 2002, I COMPLETED A 12-WEEK RESIDENTIAL HEALING JOURNEY FOR POST TRAUMATIC STRESS DISORDER AND BULIMIA. THE 'TAKE TWO' THEME WAS PERFECT IN TERMS OF MY HEALING, AND ... TO REACH OUT AND SHARE WITH OTHERS."

LYDIA KANN

OF MASSACHUSETTS HAS PUBLISHED POLITICAL COMMENTARY IN *QUEST*, AND HAS EXHIBITED WIDELY AS A VISUAL ARTIST IN NEW ENGLAND FOR THE PAST 20 YEARS. THIS IS HER FIRST PUBLISHED FICTION.

ROXANNE KAZDA

IS A CHICAGOLAND REAL ESTATE PROFESSIONAL WHO WRITES, SINGS AND ACCOMPANIES HERSELF ON THE 12-STRING GUITAR. SHE SERVES ON THE TALLGRASS BOARD OF DIRECTORS.

MARIA LOGGIA-KEE

LEARNED THE JOY OF COOKING FROM HER SICILIAN GREAT-GRANDMOTHER. AFTER WORKING FOR NEWSPAPERS AND MAGAZINES, SHE FREELANCES IN CALIFORNIA AND TEACHES AT THE COLLEGE LEVEL.

AUSTIN KELLY

ATTENDS CHICAGO'S COLUMBIA COLLEGE AS A FILM-MAKING STUDENT. HE HAS COMPLETED SEVERAL SCREENPLAYS AND SHORT STORIES. THIS IS HIS FIRST PUBLISHED FICTION.

WILFRID R. KOPONEN

PH.D., A FORMER LECTURER AT STANFORD UNIVERSITY, IS NOW SELF-EMPLOYED AS A WRITER/EDITOR IN ALBURQUERQUE. HE WON 3RD PLACE IN THE 1999 TALLGRASS WRITING CONTEST FOR FICTION.

KATHERYN K. LABORDE

OF LOUISIANA CREATED THE CHARACTERS OF JANIE LUNA AND MU BOB YANG WHILE COMPLETING HER CREATIVE WRITING DEGREE FROM THE UNIVERSITY OF NEW ORLEANS. SHE IS IN THE PROCESS OF FINISHING A NOVEL WITH JANIE AND MU BOB, AS WELL AS MU BOB'S SONGS.

C. J. LAITY

PUBLISHES ONLINE *LETTER EX*, A MAJOR RESOURCE IN CHICAGOLAND'S LITERARY COMMUNITY. THIS IMPRESARIO OF THE WRITTEN AND SPOKEN WORD ORGANIZES MAJOR POETRY READINGS INCLUDING CHICAGO'S LARGEST, POETRYFEST.

STEPHANIE JONES LAUREY

LIVES IN THE WASHINGTON, D.C. AREA WITH HER HUSBAND AND SON. SHE HAS A POEM FORTHCOMING IN *NEW ZOO POETRY REVIEW*.

MICHEL MAGEE

LIVES ON NANTUCKET ISLAND, 30 MILES TO SEA OFF THE COAST OF CAPE COD. AND HAS RECENTLY COMPLETED TWO BOOKS OF POEMS, *FALLING TOWARD HEAVEN* AND *DANCING WITH THE DEAD*. SHE IS AN AWARD-WINNING ARTIST/WRITER WHOSE NUMEROUS PUBLISHING CREDITS INCLUDE *MS. MAGAZINE*, *YANKEE*, *TRAVEL & LEISURE*, AND *NANTUCKET JOURNAL*. HER NATIONALLY AWARDED ONE-ACT PLAY, *BLUE*, IS ANTHOLOGIZED IN *MONOLOGUES FOR WOMEN BY WOMEN*.

PAMELA MALONE

OF NEW JERSEY HAS PUBLISHED HER POETRY, FICTION, AND ESSAYS IN OVER 150 MAGAZINES AND ANTHOLOGIES. HER POETRY COLLECTION, *THAT HEAVEN ONCE WAS MY HELL*, IS PUBLISHED BY LINEAR ARTS BOOKS. SHE IS THE ASSOCIATE EDITOR OF *WINGS ONLINE MAGAZINE*.

JOANNE MCFARLAND

IS A NEW YORK ARTIST/WRITER, AND AUTHOR OF THREE POETRY COLLECTIONS: *STILLS*, *BRUSHSTROKES*, AND *WATERMARKS*, AVAILABLE FROM ACORN WHISTLE PRESS.

PAMELA MILLER

IS THE AUTHOR OF *FAST LITTLE SHOES* AND *MYSTERIOUS COLESLAW*, AND HAS RECENTLY HAD POEMS PUBLISHED IN *SPOUT*, *FREE LUNCH*, AND WOMAN MADE GALLERY'S *HER MARK 2002 DATEBOOK*. BORN IN 1952, THIS CHICAGO WRITER IS CURRENTLY WORKING ON A SUITE OF POEMS CALLED *THE BODY AT FIFTY*.

FRED MUHM

OF SUBURBAN CHICAGO HAS PARTICIPATED IN MANY TALLGRASS EVENTS FOR THE LAST TWO YEARS, SERVING AS ITS IN-HOUSE SOUND ENGINEER. THIS IS HIS FIRST PUBLICATION.

CAROL A. MYERS

OF CHICAGO MAKES HER LIVING IN THE CORPORATE WORLD AS WELL AS THE CREATIVE ONE. THIS ENTREPRENEURIAL TALLGRASS MEMBER WAS A WINNER IN *A KISS IS STILL A KISS*, AND HAS BEEN PUBLISHED IN *THE POTOMAC REVIEW*.

ELLEN NORDBERG

LIVES IN SOUTHERN CALIFORNIA WHERE SHE ROCK-CLIMBS, TEACHES AEROBICS, AND EATS CARBS AND CHEESE ON OCCASION. SHE HAS HAD WORK IN *WINDY CITY SPORTS*, *ROCKY MOUNTAIN SPORTS*, *MOON JOURNAL*, SEVERAL OUTRIDER PRESS ANTHOLOGIES, AND *THE CHICAGO TRIBUNE*.

KIMBERLY G. O'LONE

OF ILLINOIS WRITES IN SEVERAL GENRES. HER WORK HAS BEEN PUBLISHED IN SEVERAL TWILIGHT TALES AND OUTRIDER PRESS ANTHOLOGIES, AND IN GIFTS FROM OUR GRANDMOTHERS, PUBLISHED BY CROWN.

LEANA PAGE

WAS BORN IN RURAL MISSISSIPPI TO A SHARECROPPING COUPLE AND NOW LIVES NEAR CHICAGO, WHERE SHE WORKS AS A TELECOMMUNICATIONS EXECUTIVE. SHE IS A GRADUATE OF ILLINOIS' ELMHURST COLLEGE WITH A B.A. IN BUSINESS ADMINISTRATION AND SOCIOLOGY. HER WORK APPEARS IN EARTH BENEATH, SKY BEYOND AND A KISS IS STILL A KISS. THIS TALLGRASS BOARD MEMBER HAS BEEN A PRINTERS ROW BOOK FAIR READER AND FEATURED READER FOR TWILIGHT TALES.

CAROLYN PAPROCKI

READS HER POETRY IN CHICAGO, WHERE SHE LIVES, WORKS, AND WRITES. SHE HAS BEEN PUBLISHED IN HAIR TRIGGER, PRINT, PUERTO DEL SOL, AND SCHOOL LIBRARY JOURNAL.

DORIS J. POPOVICH

IS A CHICAGO NATIVE AND A FRIEND TO TALLGRASS. HER WORK HAS APPEARED IN THREE PREVIOUS TALLGRASS ANTHOLOGIES, AND IN EARTH BENEATH, SKY BEYOND, SHE WON 2ND PLACE IN PROSE FOR HER NOVEL EXCERPT, "THE KINDNESS OF STRANGERS."

NANCY F. RAFAL

IS VICE PRESIDENT OF THE WISCONSIN FELLOWSHIP OF POETS AND 1/3 OF THE PERFORMANCE WRITING TRIO, "THE OFF Q GALS." THIS WISCONSIN WRITER'S WORK HAS APPEARED IN HUMMINGBIRD AND SIFTINGS.

K. S. ROSENTHAL

IS A RESIDENT PHYSICIAN AT MAINE MEDICAL CENTER IN PORTLAND. BORN IN WUPPERTAL, GERMANY, SHE LIVED IN AFRICA UNTIL SHE MOVED TO THE U.S. AT AGE SEVEN. SO FAR SHE HAS WRITTEN TWO NOVELS AND 15 SHORT STORIES.

DEBORAH DASHOW RUTH

HAS PUBLISHED IN CALIFORNIA QUARTERLY, POETS ON, COMSTOCK REVIEW, AND THE SOW'S EAR POETRY REVIEW, WHICH NOMINATED HER FOR A PUSHCART PRIZE. SHE HAS BEEN A MEMBER OF CALIFORNIA'S SQUAW VALLEY COMMUNITY OF WRITERS SINCE 1991.

LYNN VEACH SADLER

LIVES IN NORTH CAROLINA AND HAS MANY WRITING CREDITS AND AWARDS. HER FULL-LENGTH POETRY COLLECTION, MOTHERS TO THE DISAPPEARED, WAS A FINALIST IN THE 2000 BREAD LOAF WRITERS' BAKELESS PRIZE. HER STORIES HAVE WON THE NORTH CAROLINA WRITERS' NETWORK, TALUS AND SCREE, AND CREAM CITY REVIEW COMPETITIONS.

TRINIDAD SANCHEZ, JR.

IS AUTHOR OF THE BEST SELLER WHY AM I SO BROWN? HIS WORK HAS BEEN ANTHOLOGIZED IN SOULLOVELY, OPEN CITY, ART RAG, WRITTEN WITH A SPOON AND XY FILES. HE LIVES IN DENVER, WHERE HE WORKS IN THE HEAD START PROGRAM.

ROSEMARY SERLUCA

WORKS AS A TV PRODUCER, ACTOR AND WRITER. SHE HAS PUBLISHED PIECES IN SINGLE LIVING, WOMEN'S NEWS, NY SPIRIT, ON COURSE, AND THE CHRISTIAN SCIENCE MONITOR. HER ONE-ACT PLAY, BROKEN PROMISES, WAS PRODUCED AT THE THEATRE STUDIO IN NEW YORK CITY. MS. SERLUCA IS A GRADUATE OF THE N.Y.U. FILM SCHOOL AND A RECIPIENT OF A WRITING FELLOWSHIP FROM THE VIRGINIA CENTER FOR THE CREATIVE ARTS.

SHOBHA SHARMA

CAME TO THE U.S. 27 YEARS AGO WITH A DOCTORATE IN CHEMISTRY. SHE HAS LEARNED SPANISH AND NOW WORKS IN THE CHICAGO PUBLIC SCHOOLS WITH LATINO PARENTS. SHE IS FINISHING HER NOVEL ABOUT IMMIGRANT WOMEN FROM SOUTH INDIA.

BILL SHERWONIT

IS AN ALASKA-BASED NATURE WRITER WHO HAS CONTRIBUTED ARTICLES AND ESSAYS TO A VARIETY OF PUBLICATIONS. HE HAS AUTHORED SEVEN BOOKS ON ALASKA AND HAS TWO MORE IN PROGRESS. HE TEACHES A CLASS IN WILDERNESS WRITING AT THE UNIVERSITY OF ALASKA/ANCHORAGE.

VIVIAN C. SHIPLEY

EDITS CONNECTICUT REVIEW. IN 2001 SHE WON THE DANIEL VAROUJAN PRIZE FROM THE NEW ENGLAND

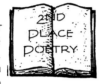

POETRY CLUB, THE CHARTER OAK REVIEW POETRY PRIZE, AND THE ROBERT FROST FOUNDATION POETRY AWARD. WHEN THERE IS NO SHORE WON THE 2002 WORD PRESS POETRY PRIZE.

KAREN KOWALSKI SINGER

OF CENTRAL ILLINOIS EDITS NEW STONE CIRCLE. HER WORK HAS APPEARED IN SLIPSTREAM, ERATICA, TIGER'S EYE, AND MY KITCHEN TABLE. 2001 AWARDS INCLUDE 2ND PLACE: SOUTHWEST WRITERS' CONTEST, AND 1ST HONORABLE MENTION: OHIO POETRY ASSOCIATION'S WINTER SOLSTICE CONTEST.

GRAZINA SMITH

OF CHICAGO HAS BEEN PUBLISHED IN PREVIOUS OUTRIDER PRESS ANTHOLOGIES AND IN KALEIDOSCOPE INK, WOMAN'S WORLD, AND CHICKEN SOUP FOR THE WOMAN'S SOUL. SHE HAS WON NATIONAL FICTION WRITING AWARDS AND IS A BOARD MEMBER OF THE TALLGRASS WRITERS GUILD.

LISA SORNBERGER

WORKS IN A PHYSICAL THERAPY DEPARTMENT FOR ADULTS WITH DEVELOPMENTAL DISABILITIES IN CONNECTICUT. HER WRITING HAS BEEN PUBLISHED IN SEVERAL LITERARY JOURNALS, AND HER AWARDS INCLUDE A 1990 FELLOWSHIP TO THE BUCKNELL SEMINAR FOR YOUNGER POETS.

RICHARD STELLA

WAS BORN IN CAMBRIDGE, MASSACHUSETTS, AND STUDIED AT NORTHEASTERN UNIVERSITY, BOSTON. HIS FOURTH CHAPBOOK, LEFTOVERS, WAS PUBLISHED IN 2001. RICHARD READS HIS POETRY THROUGHOUT THE SAN FRANCISCO BAY AREA, WHERE HE HAS LIVED FOR THE LAST 30 YEARS.

BEVERLY SWEET, R.N.

OF TEXAS HAS BEEN PUBLISHED IN SOL AND MEDHUNTERS MAGAZINES. SHE HAS BEEN A FEATURED POET IN CLEAR LAKE, TEXAS, AT BARNES & NOBLE AND THE LITERARY CLUB AT THE UNIVERSITY OF HOUSTON. SHE RECENTLY PUBLISHED HER FIRST BOOK, MIGHT BE MY HEART, AND IS AT WORK ON A SECOND.

CLAUDIA VAN GERVEN

HAS TAUGHT WRITING FOR 15 YEARS, AND HAS WORK IN PRAIRIE SCHOONER, CALYX, AND THE LULLWATER REVIEW. HER RECENTLY ANTHOLOGIZED WRITING IS IN ESSENTIAL LOVE. THIS COLORADO WRITER'S FULL-LENGTH MANUSCRIPT, THE SPIRIT STRING, WAS A BACKWATERS PRESS AND VERSE PRIZE FINALIST. HER CHAPBOOK THE ENDS OF SUNBONNET SUE WON THE 1997 ANGEL FISH PRESS AWARD.

DIANALEE VELIE

OF NEW HAMPSHIRE IS A GRADUATE OF SARAH LAWRENCE COLLEGE. SHE HAS AN M.A. IN WRITING FROM MANHATTANVILLE COLLEGE, WHERE SHE SERVED AS FACULTY ADVISOR OF INKWELL MAGAZINE, THE LITERARY JOURNAL OF THE MAW PROGRAM, AND TAUGHT THE CRAFT OF WRITING. SHE TEACHES COURSES IN POETRY AND MEMOIR AT DARTMOUTH COLLEGE, AND HER POETRY WORKSHOPS, BELDEN ISLAND MAGIC, CONTINUE TO SELL OUT. HER WORK IS IN HUNDREDS OF LITERARY JOURNALS THROUGHOUT THE U.S. AND CANADA; THEY INCLUDE KALLIOPE, THE POTOMAC REVIEW, AND THE SOUTH DAKOTA REVIEW.

KEVIN WATSON WAS BORN IN ILLINOIS A N D RAISED IN

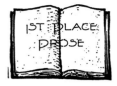

MISSOURI. HE NOW LIVES WITH HIS WIFE AND CHILDREN IN WINSTON-SALEM, NORTH CAROLINA, AND IS A STUDENT AT SALEM COLLEGE (AMERICA'S OLDEST ALL-WOMAN'S COLLEGE, EST. 1772), WHERE HE IS A PROUD "SALEM SISTER." EARNING HIS DEGREE IN ENGLISH AND CREATIVE WRITING. HIS STORIES HAVE APPEARED IN *ART IDEAS MAGAZINE, THE ROSE & THORN, AMARILLO BAY,* AND OTHERS.

ANTHONY RUSSELL WHITE

WRITES, " I AM A PILGRIM, A POET, AND A HEALER. I LIVE ON A MOUNTAIN TOP IN SAN RAFAEL, CALIFORNIA, AND SERVE ON THE PERMANENT STAFF OF THE NINE GATES MYSTERY SCHOOL. I HAVE BEEN WRITING POETRY (AGAIN) SINCE 1992. MAJOR INFLUENCES HAVE BEEN WILLIAM STAFFORD, ROBERT BLY, AND OF COURSE, RUMI."

TAMMY WILSON

HAS SHORT FICTION IN *BIG MUDDY, NORTH CAROLINA LITERARY REVIEW* AND KAY ALLENBAUGH'S *CHOCOLATE* SERIES. SHE HAS WORKED AS A PR DIRECTOR IN NORTH CAROLINA, WHERE MUCH OF HER WORK IS SET. SHE COMPLETES HER SECOND FICTION WRITING RESIDENCY AT VERMONT STUDIO CENTER IN 2002.

DAN WITTE

HAS HAD FICTION PUBLISHED IN PREVIOUS "BLACK-AND-WHITE" ANTHOLOGIES, WINNING 1ST PLACE IN THE 2000 PROSE CATEGORY. WORK BY THIS CHICAGO-AREA WRITER HAS ALSO APPEARED IN *THE HIGH PLAINS LITERARY REVIEW,* WHERE HE HAS BEEN TWICE NOMINATED FOR A PUSHCART PRIZE.

MARGARET YOUNG

OF OBERLIN, OHIO HAS HAD HER POEMS AND ESSAYS PUBLISHED IN NUMEROUS LITERARY MAGAZINES, AND IS CURRENTLY WORKING ON A NOVEL. HER FIRST BOOK OF POETRY, RECENTLY PUBLISHED BY CLEVELAND STATE UNIVERSITY PRESS, IS *WILLOW FROM THE WILLOW.* SHE EARNED DEGREES FROM YALE UNIVERSITY AND UNIVERSITY OF CALIFORNIA/DAVIS, WORKED IN A TRAVELING THEATER COMPANY, AND TAUGHT CREATIVE WRITING AT ALLEGHANY COLLEGE.

PEGGY ZABICKI

ATTENDED ST. XAVIER UNIVERSITY IN CHICAGO, WHERE SHE WRITES AND LIVES WITH HER HUSBAND AND FOUR CHILDREN. SHE WORKS IN RETAIL DURING THE DAY AND TUTORS CHILDREN IN READING AT NIGHT. ON DAYS OFF SHE WRITES "ABOUT THINGS I KNOW AND

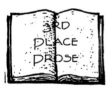

PLACES I'VE NEVER BEEN." HER WINNING STORY, "TWINKIE DREAMS," IS HER FIRST NATIONAL PUBLICATION.

hitney Scott plays many roles in Chicago's literary scene. She is an author, editor, book designer and reviewer whose poetry, fiction and creative non-fiction have been published internationally, earning her listings in *Contemporary Authors* and *Directory of American Poets and Fiction Writers.* Her work has appeared in respected reviews and journals, including *Howling Dog, Kaleidoscope Ink, Pearl, Potomac Review, Art & Understanding, Amethyst, CQ, The Poetry Peddler, Arts Alive, Dangerous Dames, The F.O.C. Review, Tomorrow Magazine, After Hours,* and others.

She performs her work at colleges, universities, arts festivals and literary venues throughout the Chicago area and has been featured as guest author in the Illinois Authors Series at Chicago's Harold Washington Library. Scott regularly reviews books for the American Library Association's *Booklist* magazine.

In addition to working one-on-one with developing writers, Whitney runs a variety of writers' workshops and has headlined the Taste of Chicago Writers conference. She has presented writing seminars at DePaul and Northwestern Universities and taught poetry workshops at the renowned Off-Campus Writers Workshop. Whitney teaches at Columbia College/Chicago.

im W. Brown, judge of the Poetry division, is well known in and beyond Chicago's literary scene. Formerly the editor of *Tomorrow Magazine,* he is the author of three novels: *Left of the Loop* (2001), *Deconstruction Acres* (1997), and the recently completed *Walking Man.* His poetry, fiction, and non-fiction have appeared in over 200 publications.

ark Knoblauch, judge of the Prose division, worked for 26 years in acquisitions and collection management for Chicago Public Library. He was also the esteemed restaurant crtitic of *The Chicago Tribune* for 15 years. He writes "Cuisine du Jour" reviews of current books on food and wine for the American Library Association's *Booklist* magazine.

ABOUT TALLGRASS WRITERS GUILD

allGrass Writers Guild is open to all who write seriously at any level, whether writing little or much, for publication or not. The Guild supports members by providing performance and publication opportunities via its six-page, bi-monthly newsletter, open mikes, formal readings, annual anthologies, and the TallGrass Writers Guild Performance Ensemble programs.

In affiliation with Outrider Press, TallGrass produces an annual anthology, the result of an international call for entries. Cash prizes and certificates are awarded, resulting from the decisions of independent judges.

The Guild is a rarity among arts organizations in that it neither seeks nor accepts federal funding because of the creative limitations imposed by such grants, often of an arbitrary and political nature. TallGrass is an independent, self-supporting organization striving to keep the First Amendment strong. While other groups have reduced programming or disappeared altogether due to cutbacks in government funding, the Guild has grown and flourished in the last 10 years, expanding the services and support it provides writers everywhere. For information on TallGrass membership and programs, call 708-672-6630 or call toll-free at 1-800-933-4680 (code 03). Visit the "Publishing" section of the Outrider Press website at www.outriderpress.com for additional details on the TallGrass Writers Guild.

Outrider Press Publications

A Kiss Is Still A Kiss – *$16.95*   _____
Writings on romantic love

Earth Beneath, Sky Beyond – *$16.95*   _____
An anthology on nature and our planet

Feathers, Fins & Fur – *$15.95*   _____
Poetry, short fiction and creative non-fiction on animals

Freedom's Just Another Word – *$14.95*   _____
Poetry, fiction and essays: international authors on freedom

Alternatives: Roads Less Travelled – *$14.95*   _____
International writings on counter-culture life-styles

Prairie Hearts – *$14.95*   _____
Short fiction and poetry on the Heartland

Dancing to the End of the Shining Bar – *$9.95*   _____
A novel of love and courage

Listen to the Moon – *$4.00*   _____
Poetry of family love and loss

Illinois residents add 8.5% [.085] sales tax   _____
Add shipping charges:
  $2.95 for one book   _____
  $4.95 for two books   _____
  $1.25 for each additional book   _____

Total   _____

Send Check or Money Order to:
Outrider Press, Inc.
937 Patricia
Crete, IL 60417

www.outriderpress.com
outriderpr@aol.com